It Happened to Me

Series Editor: Arlene Hirschfelder

Books in the It Happened To Me series are designed for inquisitive teens digging for answers about certain illnesses, social issues, or lifestyle interests. Whether you are deep into your teen years or just entering them, these books are gold mines of up-to-date information, riveting teen views, and great visuals to help you figure out stuff. Besides special boxes highlighting singular facts, each book is enhanced with the latest reading list, websites, and an index. Perfect for browsing, there's loads of expert information by acclaimed writers to help parents, guardians, and librarians understand teen illness, tough situations, and lifestyle choices.

1. *Learning Disabilities: The Ultimate Teen Guide,* by Penny Hutchins Paquette and Cheryl Gerson Tuttle, 2003.
2. *Epilepsy: The Ultimate Teen Guide,* by Kathlyn Gay and Sean McGarrahan, 2002.
3. *Stress Relief: The Ultimate Teen Guide,* by Mark Powell, 2002.
4. *Making Sexual Decisions: The Ultimate Teen Guide,* by L. Kris Gowen, Ph.D., 2003.
5. *Asthma: The Ultimate Teen Guide,* by Penny Hutchins Paquette, 2003.
6. *Cultural Diversity: Conflicts and Challenges: The Ultimate Teen Guide,* by Kathlyn Gay, 2003.
7. *Diabetes: The Ultimate Teen Guide,* by Katherine J. Moran, 2004.
8. *When Will I Stop Hurting? Teens, Loss, and Grief: The Ultimate Teen Guide,* by Edward Myers, 2004.
9. *Volunteering: The Ultimate Teen Guide,* by Kathlyn Gay, 2004.
10. *Organ Transplants: A Survival Guide for The Entire Family: The Ultimate Teen Guide,* by Tina P. Schwartz, 2005.
11. *Medications: The Ultimate Teen Guide,* by Cheryl Gerson Tuttle, 2005.

Organ Transplants

A Survival Guide for The Entire Family: The Ultimate Teen Guide

TINA P. SCHWARTZ

It Happened to Me, No. 10

The Scarecrow Press, Inc.
Lanham, Maryland • Toronto • Oxford
2005

SCARECROW PRESS, INC.

Published in the United States of America
by Scarecrow Press, Inc.
A wholly owned subsidary of
The Rowman & Littlefield Publishing Group, Inc.
4501 Forbes Boulevard, Suite 200, Lanham, Maryland 20706
www.scarecrowpress.com

PO Box 317
Oxford
OX2 9RU, UK

British Library Cataloguing in Publication Information Available

Library of Congress Cataloging-in-Publication Data

Schwartz, Tina P., 1969–
  Organ transplants : a survival guide for the entire family : the ultimate teen guide / Tina P. Schwartz.
      p. cm. — (It happened to me ; no. 10)
  Includes bibliographical references and index.
  ISBN 0-8108-4924-0 (alk. paper)
  1. Transplantation of organs, tissues, etc.—Popular works. I. Title. II. Series.
RD120.75.S38 2005
617.9'5—dc22

                                                            2004021563

For my dad . . . Jim Purcell

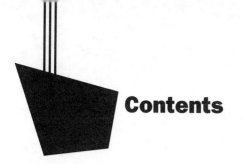

Contents

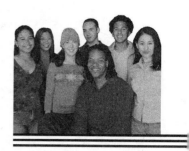

Contents

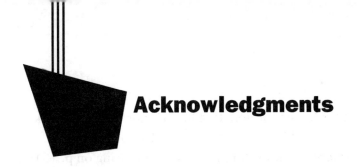

Acknowledgments

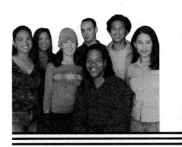

There are so many people to thank for helping me write this book. I start with my dad and mom, Jim and Diane Purcell; my husband Marc and children, Cameron, Heather, and Brandon; along with my entire family and friends, whose love and support make my life possible. I thank God for you all every day.

Next, are the people who answered the countless numbers of questions I had; forgive me if I've forgotten anyone. They gave me permission to use information from their websites and phone interviews I had with them, not to mention numerous e-mails: first and foremost, Joel Newman, from the United Network for Organ Sharing (UNOS). Joel is the most thorough, swift, and professional person you could work with. He is exactly the person you want handling details of an organization like UNOS, where life and death is at stake. Thank you for being such a tremendous help!

Thanks go to Kim McCullough and Kate Pianetto, both from Gift of Hope Organ and Tissue Donor Network, who also survived my many e-mails and phone calls with endless questions; Gwendolyn Maddox from the National Minority Organ Tissue and Transplant Education Program (MOTTEP); Kathy Dasgupta, University of Chicago Hospital; Jacqueline Key at the Gale Group; Marie Elebash at Kid Kare; Reg Green at the Nicholas Green Foundation; Charley Parker for donating his "Donorsaurs" artwork, courtesy of Gift of Life Donor Program, www.donors1.org, on pp. 21, 39, 47, 143, 156, and 206; DiNanno Photography for permission to use the photo on

Acknowledgments

pp. 109; Brent Moats for donating his "Donor Man" artwork, courtesy of Gift of Hope Organ & Tissue Donor Network, www.giftofhope.org/kids/donorman.asp, appearing on p. 151; Frank Bodino from the Transplant-Speakers International; and the Transplant Recipients International Organization, Inc. (TRIO). Thanks also to John Baer (of Sonnenshein, Nath and Rosenthal) for his legal expertise.

Thanks also to the participants and their families for sharing their personal experiences: Linda Bowers, Crystal Capser, Michelle and Ed Eymer, Judith Fringuello, Dave Goodwin, Reg Green, Jim Leman, Celeste Morris, the Namowicz family, Jim Purcell, Alan Raskin, and Stoney Weiszmann.

Professionally and personally I thank Anne Courtright whose countless hours of editing, pep talks and FrappuccinosTM made the sometimes lonely job of writing quite festive. And thank you for your beautiful artwork on pages 27, 50, 62, 65, and 81. What a fabulous contribution. Thank you to Conrad Locander (a.k.a. Professor Whimsey), my other brilliant artist and friend whose creatures created especially for this book creatures created especially for this book (on pp. 1, 13, 25, 43, 59, 77, 99, 113, 131, 141, 159, 183, and 197), gave it true personality. Thanks to all my SCBWI friends (the Society of Children's Book Writers and Illustrators), especially my critique group buddies (Anne, Hal, Lorijo, Denise, Laurie, and Shawn), and to my regional advisor Esther Hirshenhorn. A special thanks to my writing mentor Melanie Apel, whose help, friendship, and support are immeasurable.

Last, and most important, thanks to Arlene Hirschfelder, the most wonderful editor a girl could have! You took a chance on an unknown author and believed in my passion and vision. Your unending supply of articles and tidbits made a wonderful contribution and proved what I suspected from the start, you are the most well-read person I've ever met.

Thank you all from the bottom of my heart.

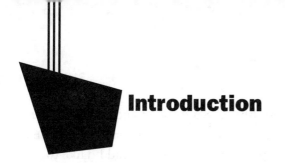

Introduction

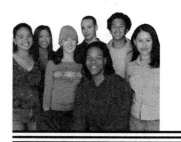

When I was in my 20s, my dad had a liver transplant. The whole ordeal, including the years that lead up to it, and afterward as well, was a life-changing experience with an inexplicable range of emotions. Unfortunately, it is a life lesson that you can only fully understand by living through it. I'm sorry that you find yourself needing this book, but remember, it is a good thing that someone you love is trying for a new chance at life.

When my dad was first told he needed a transplant, I looked and looked for books addressing family members, one that targeted me specifically. I wanted something to answer questions that I couldn't ask out loud. Although I am the youngest of five children, I felt uncomfortable saying certain things to my brothers and sisters. Even though we are a close family, I was afraid to utter that one question out loud: "What if he dies?" I imagine most everyone in the family probably thought it, but I don't remember us talking about it.

There are some great books out there for organ recipients, and sometimes even a chapter or so for spouses. However, I was frustrated to find—or rather *not* find—a book specifically for family members.

I also want to address the donors and their families. For without them, we'd all be lost!

I hope this book helps to relieve some fears, answer some questions you might be having, and help to put your mind at ease.

The beginning of adulthood is a difficult and stressful time in a person's life, even under the best of circumstances. I hope it helps to hear other people share their stories; and I'd like to thank them for their honesty and bravery in opening up their hearts to share with us.

Best wishes to you and your family. Remember you are *not* alone!

DISCLAIMER

None of the medical information in this book is meant to replace the advice of doctors. This information is intended as a reference for family members eager to learn about transplants and emotional issues that arise from going through similar experiences. Some of the quotes in this book are from people who wanted their names changed to protect their privacy.

1 Getting the News

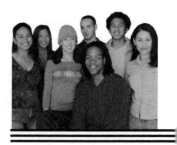

"He needs a transplant? Are you joking? I don't believe it. I know you see and hear about transplants all the time now on TV and in movies. Even when you get your driver's license, they ask if you want to sign a donor card. But jeez! You never really think something so extreme and weird could happen in your own family. How are my parents going to handle this? How am I going to deal with this? Will my dad die? This is too huge!" That's how I felt when I learned my dad needed a liver transplant.

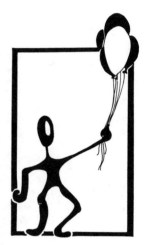

> A young man named Bud said, "I was so scared for my father. I needed to know how serious this was, how immediate. When would he actually need a transplant? Would he be on the list for years? Would he survive if he had to wait too long?"

Other young adults were happy to learn their parent was on the transplant waiting list. George, who was 17 years old when his mom told him she needed a transplant, said, "I was excited for her to get a [lung] transplant, once I knew that the success rate was high. My mom had trouble walking and trouble getting ready on her own. My biggest concern was, could she die in surgery?"

George's sister Annie, who was 23 at the time of surgery and also living away from home, said, "My mom let me know she went on a list but that she thought it would be a while before a donor came around for her to get the lungs, so not to worry. I asked her questions as she received material about transplants, but at the same time, I did not see this as a reality that she was getting a transplant, so I tried to forget about it in the back of my mind."

Annie went on to say, "I asked questions like how long will you be in the hospital? Will you definitely live through the surgery? What are the odds of you dying? Will this cure your emphysema? [Looking back now, after her surgery] I was ignorant to what the process included . . . my mom did not really tell me much, not to the extent of what I should have been told. Now I wonder why we did not take the pretransplant process as seriously as we should have."

HOW IT ALL STARTS

Reality check: When the moment finally comes for your parent to be put on the United Network for Organ Sharing (UNOS) list, it makes every fear come true. I believe the majority of people must be in denial until their parent is actually on the list.

My family said, "Yeah, we knew it was coming," but I believe in my heart most of us were still shocked when it became official.

Personally, I thought, "What? I didn't know it was coming!" I don't know how I could have blanked out such a huge problem, but I swear I knew nothing of it prior to the word *transplant* coming up when my dad had decided to have his name put on the list.

By the time someone is sick enough for a transplant, most of the family knows and expects it. For some reason, I was totally in shock. Granted, I am the biggest optimist on the planet, but I did not see this coming. Here's how it plays out in some families:

1. **Person gets sick.**

2. **Person is ill for years.**

3. **No medications or procedures will prolong life (i.e., been on dialysis too long; or is on oxygen full time).**

4. **Transplant is only chance for survival.**

5. **All avenues exhausted:**

   ◎ **No relatives have matching tissues/blood type/etc. needed to become a donor; or it's a nonoption if heart is needed (versus a kidney, which can come from a living donor).**

   ◎ **Other organs start shutting down because of the stress the illness has put on the rest of the body.**

   ◎ **Person gets placed on a list of patients waiting for an organ (or multiple organ) transplant. In the United States, the list is from the UNOS.**

6. **Doctors give an estimate of how long your parent has to live without a transplant.**

7. **Patient gradually moves up the list with each illness.**

8. **Patient finally becomes sick enough to get a pager.**

> A young woman named Hannah said, "I knew a transplant was inevitable, but I was still pretty horrified when it became official that she [her aunt] would actually be put on the official UNOS (United Network for Organ Sharing) list."

   ◎ **Illness becomes tricky since a potential recipient cannot be sick when an organ becomes available (if patient has a bad cold or fever, the transplant team may decide not to operate because the patient will have a compromised immune system after surgery).**

   ◎ **Age can play a factor, although that is an "unwritten rule."[1] Transplants are not simply to prolong life but to enhance it. With donor organs in such huge demand and fatally short supply, doctors in the transplant community want to be sure all organs available go to people who will get the greatest use from them.**

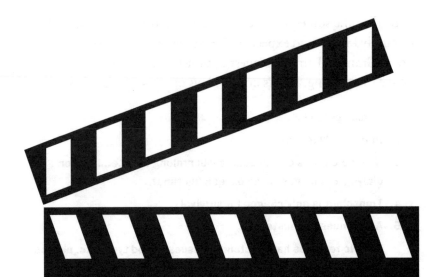

CHECK AND RECHECK

In the movie *John Q* (New Line Productions, 2002) starring Denzel Washington, when a couple's son collapses at his little league game, they discover he'll need a heart transplant to survive. Although both parents work, their health insurance policy will not cover a procedure that large because of a technicality.

The movie focuses on the debate about health insurance coverage. The father is an hourly employee in a bad economy with business slowing down. When his hours get cut, he is given a smaller health insurance policy. The issue is that the family's coverage is changed without written notification to them, and the premiums are still being deducted from each paycheck. Also, as a result of the smaller policy, the child's name is not able to be added on the national recipient waiting list without a $50,000 cash down payment (20% of a $250,000 operation).

Contributions from friends, family, the church community, plus selling everything they have of value (like their car, TV, engagement and wedding rings) only amount to $22,000. The hospital says it is very strict about cash accounts and down payments. The family will need to come up with the additional $28,000 before the son's name can be added to the list.

◎ Certain organs, but not all, can be considered for transplantation in cancer patients.[2] Former football great Walter Payton, who had cancer, needed a liver transplant. By the time he was high enough on the transplant list, it was too late to save his life. His cancer had progressed too far.

INSURANCE PROBLEM HITS HOME

My father checked with his insurance company numerous times to be sure his policy would cover a liver transplant. It was one of the very first things on his "to do" list. They assured him repeatedly that he was indeed covered. After much testing and getting him ready to be put on the UNOS list, someone finally discovered that, in fact, he was *not* covered for the procedure. Technically, they would cover *treatment* necessary for managing his illness, Hepatitis C, but would not cover an actual procedure as large as a transplant. After a certain amount of time, though, a transplant is the only option left for "treatment."

The situation in the movie *John Q* shows a realistic problem people face today, when a family has no insurance or has a policy that doesn't cover catastrophic illnesses or procedures such as transplants. It is important for your family to check and recheck that insurance will not be an issue.

Luckily, my dad was able to continue on his own insurance policy through his work before it lapsed. He was transferring to my mom's insurance plan because they thought the coverage would be better. If he hadn't been able to stay on his own policy, our family would have had to raise the money for the nearly $500,000 operation. Some of my siblings wondered whether they should cash in their kids' college funds and/or mortgage their houses. Because I still lived with my parents, I wasn't much help financially. I could only hope my being there provided some emotional support during the agonizing wait.

DO YOUR HOMEWORK . . . DO SOME RESEARCH

When talking about "getting on the UNOS list," most people don't realize 11 regions are in the country; each are like subunits of the national waiting list.[3] Waiting recipients should research each region's guidelines to determine which one might give them a better chance to get the organ they need in the time the doctors estimate they have left to live. It is not easy, or even sometimes possible, to do this. Chicago, for example, has one of the leading liver transplant centers in the country (at University of Chicago Hospital).

This type of information might bring up a discussion about the value of moving. Because my dad needed a liver, and we lived in the suburbs of Chicago, we already lived in a great place to help his particular needs.

Although some places perform more transplants (Florida has three or four centers, where North Dakota has none), that doesn't mean waiting recipients will get a transplant quicker living in Florida. The centers work on a population basis, so if there are less people who live in an area, statistically there will be fewer organs available, too. If you calculate the percentages, it might work out the same by staying near your house or going to another region. Your parent and family must decide whether it is truly worth it to shake up your world even more by moving.

CRAZY IDEA, OR NOT?

Moving to another "region" is an extreme idea that would need to be a family decision. Everyone's situation should be evaluated. One of the lung recipients who is highlighted in Chapter 6 (Celeste Morris) was going to move to St. Louis (from the suburbs of Chicago). As it turns out, the waiting list for lung transplants was much longer at Barnes Jewish Hospital in St. Louis than the one at Loyola University Medical Center in Chicago. She also wasn't sure if she would be covered by insurance at Loyola. Luckily, she was covered by insurance at Loyola, so she didn't have to move.

If she had decided to go to St. Louis, she would have gotten a call when her doctors estimated she had approximately 3 months

A young adult named Lisa said she was embarrassed to admit it, but she couldn't help thinking, "What about me? My dad cosigned a loan for my brother's first car. He walked my sisters down the aisle when they got married. He saw my brothers and sisters become parents. I'm only in high school. At this rate, I'll be lucky if he makes it to my graduation!"

left until she moved to the top of the list. Then she and her family would move to St. Louis. A huge decision like that can disrupt an entire family. Not that everyone would *have* to go with her, but she would need some support system there while waiting.

If this happened the summer before your senior year of high school, your parents would probably not want to move you and your family. Because the wait time is so unknown, you need to keep your life as "normal" as possible within the entire family.

Many people don't realize that there are no standard guidelines that each region has to follow. No uniformity is required. Critics feel that each of the 11 regions must decide the main function of its registry. Some examples of these functions would be to increase the number of donors, help make the consent to donate easier, and increase public awareness and education. One of the states recognized for its innovative and effective state registry programs is Pennsylvania.

Another idea to help connect the country in the transplant effort is to develop computer registries for interstate linkage and 24-hour access. But things like standardizing donor registries, adding computer registries, and other "big ideas" will cost tons of money. Money will have to be budgeted by the Federal Government if such a huge undertaking is going to happen. It would be impossible for private investors to do alone.

THE STARS NEED TO PRACTICALLY ALIGN!

Getting a transplant involves so many pieces falling into place at one time that it is amazing anyone ever receives a transplant! Luckily, transplants *do* happen every day now. Here is what needs to happen:

- **Transplant coordinator tells patient he or she is officially on the UNOS waiting list and will receive written confirmation as well (but from the coordinator, not from UNOS).**
- **Because of the shortage of organs, the wait time on the UNOS list can be a mysterious and stressful time. There is no way to predict how long a person will be on the list. Some people get a transplant before receiving a pager, while others are on the list indefinitely.**

Waiting List	**87,328 as of**
Candidates	**12/17/04**
Transplants	**20,303 as of**
	Jan.–Sep. 2004
Donors	**10,603[4] as of**
	Jan.–Sep. 2004

- Once a donor is found, the organ must be successfully procured, or removed, without any errors. The slightest nick could damage the organ and render it useless.

- Blood type, tissue compatibility, and a series of other tests must be performed to find the perfect match. Things to help a match considered perfect might include height, body frame, and even nationality.

- When the proper recipient is chosen and contacted, he or she must be in good health and within a certain driving distance of the hospital.

- The organ must get to the correct transplant center safely and in a timely manner. Each organ has a certain life span once removed from a person. Some expire within hours.[5]

After reading all that needs to happen, it is amazing that many transplants happen in the United States each and every day. Keep that in mind when you're starting to feel that it's hopeless. Hope is a *huge* commodity that you cannot afford to give away!

FOLLOW YOUR DOCTOR OR YOUR HOSPITAL?

My dad was originally set to go to a hospital called Rush-Presbyterian-St. Luke's, also in Chicago, until the whole insurance fiasco happened. He had to change hospitals if he wanted insurance coverage, so that decision was an easy one.

However, another person I spoke with chose to follow his doctors when they changed hospitals. On some HMO plans, you follow a doctor or practice, not a hospital. My dad had to get

HOW TO REDUCE STRESS WHILE WAITING FOR TRANSPLANT:

Talk to someone: Whether it's a friend or family member, talk about what scares you or is stressing you out. You can even call the transplant coordinator who can put you in touch with a social worker, counselor, or local support group if you don't want to talk to people you know about personal stuff. The waiting period will probably be the hardest time for you.

Exercise: It is a great way to burn off stress and clear your mind. Plus, it is best for everyone to stay as healthy as possible. Tons of stress can wear you down and lower your immunity. The last thing you need to do is get a cold or the flu; or even risk giving it to your parent and wreck his or her chance to have surgery if the call should come.

Have a Plan of Where You'll Stay: You or your parent will be called away and have to leave immediately. Depending on your age, you can even ask a friend to be your point-person for somewhere to stay for a few days while your parent is getting the transplant. This will help your parents out by not having to worry about you. Plus, even if you're in your late teens, you shouldn't be alone at such a scary time. You'll probably spend a lot of time at the hospital, but at nighttime, it will help to be with someone you feel close to.

Tie Up Loose Ends: You might want to write a letter to your parent ahead of time and just keep it in an envelope. You can seal it and have them read it when you are the one having surgery, or pack it in the bag your parent has ready for the hospital if he or she is the one having the surgery. Your parent will have it to read as he or she goes to the hospital.

It's really hard to say all the things you want to a person, especially when you're face to face. When I actually saw my father wheeled away to surgery and realized that I may never see him again, there were things I wondered if he knew (See poem in Chapter 8).

new doctors at the new hospital since the team he had been with for years had privileges to practice at his old hospital, but not the new one.

The medical team change was an adjustment for my dad because he had dealt with the same doctors and support staff over several years prior to the change. Forming a new trust would take some time. Your parent needs to trust the team completely since his or her life is literally in the doctors and nurses hands. The right doctor-patient bond can give your family, and parent, a comfort level to be able to go through with an organ transplant.

YOUR ROLE IS IMPORTANT

For people to be considered for transplantation, a very important factor is their support system. Before patients can be put on the list, they need to show they have people in their lives to help them manage their care and keep their spirits up. Recovery will be a long haul, full of peaks and valleys. One of the biggest hurdles people face that others don't realize is the depression that will go along with the whole situation, even posttransplant. Whether you are the one having the transplant or not, you play an important part in the entire process.

Getting used to all the medications is overwhelming. Recipients often feel that their whole lives are just about keeping schedules of their medications and what to take when. I remember in the first few months after my dad's transplant, he was sitting at the kitchen table with his shoulders slumped down and said, "Is this it? Is this all my life is going to be, just figuring out what medicine to take when? I'll never keep it all straight."

Before surgery, you and your parent can make a big three-ring binder together to help keep you or him or her organized after the transplant. You can put in various tabs like "Current Medications" that says what you or he or she is taking (pre- and posttransplant), what each medicine is for (what it is supposed to do), the dosage, any reactions to it, and so forth.

Another tab can be for "Follow-up Visits." It can have a chart for each doctor or physical therapy session, and so on. You can make it less "sterile" or boring by putting in pictures every few pages, stickers, encouraging notes, or whatever you think will help put a smile on your or your parent's face. Plus, doing it together will make you both feel like a team, like you each aren't in this situation "alone."

There is a huge adjustment period for everyone, starting from the recipient feeling lousy, to family members being sick of the person being crabby all the time. My father took a lot of things in stride his whole life, and after his transplant it seemed like he couldn't tolerate anything. If someone did something to bug him, he would just blow up at the person. Years later, he's not as emotional anymore, yet he has never quite gone back to being so passive, either.

There may be times when you or your parent get really upset about seemingly minor things. Others might look at you and think, "Who are you? Are you seriously having a total cow over *this*?" Don't worry, the edginess will eventually diminish. You won't always feel like you're on an emotional roller coaster!

Because I can't even imagine the range of emotions my dad, or any recipient, has to deal with on a daily basis, it sounds horrible and petty of me to even mention these temper flare-ups. But I do this so you don't feel so alone if this happens in your family. It is not uncommon. Give yourself a break and stop thinking of yourself as mean for being sick of your parent being crabby or on edge or complaining a lot. Consider if you were given a second chance at life, you might want to do things differently. In my dad's case, he became much more assertive and adopted a type of "zero tolerance" for anything that irritates him. After years of letting most everything roll off his back, or just holding things in, I don't feel too badly that he now makes more of his feelings known. I think it may be healthier for him in the long run; no more ulcers!

ONE THOUSAND TIMES, THANK YOU, BUT CAN I GET ON WITH MY LIFE NOW?

Transplant patients may eventually get tired of always having to feel grateful. Of course they are happy to be alive and amazingly, indescribably grateful for their gift of life. At some point it cannot be the entire focus of their lives. They need to return to some normalcy. Life cannot always revolve around "the transplant."

It sounds horrible, but is touched on so well in the movie *Return to Me* (Metro-Goldwyn-Mayer Pictures, 2000) with David Duchovny and Minnie Driver. Minnie's character (Grace) gets a heart transplant and, a year after the surgery, is having a depressed moment during a doctor's visit. She confesses to the doctor that she feels guilty for being depressed when she knows she should be happy. These mixed emotions are quite common for recipients, especially those who received organs from someone who died.

In that same scene, Grace is about to go on talking about her feelings when the doctor makes some totally unrelated comment, showing he is not listening to her at all. It paints a very bleak picture for the bedside manner of some doctors. Luckily, all doctors are not really like that, although some tend to be a bit dry.

Later in the movie, Grace's grandfather, played by Carol O'Connor, tells her to visit a church to thank the saints. The grandfather's friend tells the grandpa to leave her alone, that she's been plenty grateful and to just let her live! *That is a sentiment that recipients cannot hear enough.* Of course you're grateful, but your life must go on. You had a life before the transplant, now you have one after as well.

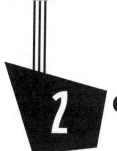

General Info to Know

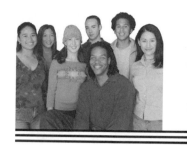

The point of this chapter is to give you a quick "crash course" on some questions you may have and terms you may be hearing. Instead of feeling like you're hearing a foreign language, this will help you follow conversations between doctors and your parents, or even doctors speaking directly to you regarding your parent's or your own health.

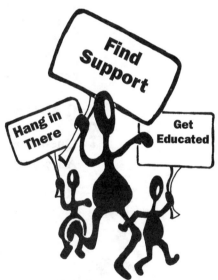

If you want more specific information about a certain transplant, then move on to individual chapters (i.e., lung, liver, kidney/pancreas, heart) but this chapter is a great beginning to get familiar with terms you'll hear, no matter what organ is being transplanted.

Something about being informed always takes a bit of the scariness out of a situation. Not that you or your parent, or even a friend going through this, become well after learning more info, but conquering your fear of the unknown can really help. It's just like the old "monster under the bed" feeling you got in the middle of the night when you were little. Once you turned on the light to see no one was there, you could fall back to sleep a lot easier than if your mind kept racing as you imagined the most horrible creatures ever.

You might have some questions that don't appear in these chapters, for example, on uncommon transplants, like intestines, hands, stomachs, etc. If you're not sure where to look for certain topics, then this "general chapter" is probably the right spot to start reading. Of course, you can always flip to the Index or the Glossary in the back of the book to help you search, too.

QUESTION: WHAT TYPE OF TRANSPLANT DOES NOT REQUIRE TISSUE TYPING, LIKE MATCHING UP BLOOD TYPE, ETC?

Answer: Corneal transplants do not need tissue typing because corneas do not have their own blood supply. This greatly reduces the chance that immune cells will come in contact with the cornea and recognize it as foreign. Therefore, corneas can be transplanted from any person to any person with little chance of rejection.[1]

Q AND A: RANDOM QUESTIONS ANSWERED

? Question:
Are stomach transplants performed?

Answer:

Some people's stomachs do not work, and they get fed through a tube instead of eating. Although that is a huge life adjustment because eating seems to be a big part of American culture, in terms of socializing, the stomach is not responsive to transplantation. It sounds weird, but it is possible to survive and lead a relatively normal life without a stomach. In fact, famous stock car driver Richard Petty had his stomach removed.[2]

? Question:
Are large intestines transplanted?

Answer:
"The large intestine is not necessary to sustain life, so it is not usually transplanted. The small intestine is also not absolutely necessary for life since intravenous feeding can take the place of the absorption of food and fluid from the intestine. This treatment is called *total parenteral nutrition (TPN)*. However,

TPN can result in liver disease in some patients. These patients then need either a small bowel transplant or a combined liver/small bowel transplant. The large intestine has been transplanted in some rare circumstances, but only in conjunction with the small intestine. This practice has been abandoned however, because the risk of infection was too high."[3]

?

Question:

My parents have been so nasty to each other lately, will they get divorced because of this whole transplant business?

Answer:

Not everyone's spouse is a saint. Many are far from it and the transplant, or waiting for it, might bring out the really nasty side of a partner. Perhaps selfishness comes through as a defense mechanism to "harden the heart" in case the person should actually die of the illness before getting surgery.

Maybe the healthy person is just sick of everyone always asking about how his or her spouse, or even teen, is doing and never stopping to think how that person is doing throughout the ordeal. If it's you that is getting the transplant, perhaps your parents are just so worried sick about you that they are pushing everyone they care about away.

No matter what the reason, if your parents fight a ton now, or you find yourself constantly battling with your parent, try not to feel guilty.

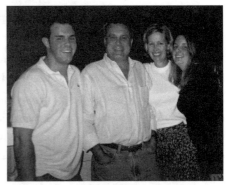

Celeste Morris with husband George and children George and Annie

"Try to have your s–t together when it happens because if you don't, it will be one million times harder when it [the transplant] happens. Also, find out everything you can about the transplant [beforehand]. That makes you a little bit more comfortable," advises George, 19 years old, whose mom had a double-lung transplant.

Every family goes through some stress. It's unavoidable. Tough situations tend to bring people closer together or pull them apart. People rarely just stay the same as always—especially with life-threatening circumstances like your family is experiencing.

It might take a while for the bickering to stop but hang in there. You can get through it together, one step at a time. Don't lose hope.

? Question:

How do I know if I really need to be on the national transpant waiting list or not? And how do I get on it?

Answer:

There are five basic steps to take to see if you are ready to be put on the UNOS waiting list, and how to go about getting on the list:

1. **There are over 200 transplant hospitals around the country. Look into ones that are close to your home first, that handle the type of transplant you need, then contact those hospitals to be sure you meet their criteria for accepting patients.**

2. **Make an appointment to get an evaluation with the transplant team at the hospital you have chosen.**

3. **During the evaluation, come prepared with as many questions as you can think of. This will be your prime opportunity to learn everything possible about the specific hospital, transplant team, history, successes in the field, and so forth. After all, you are essentially interviewing *them* as well.**

4. **The hospital's transplant team will decide whether you are a good candidate for its program. Since each hospital has its own criteria for accepting patients, some will take you and some might not.**

5. **If the team at the hospital decides you will be a good candidate for them, they will add you to the UNOS national waiting list.[4]**

? Question:

How do I know for sure if and when I am officially on "the list"?

Answer:

UNOS does *not* send patients written confirmation of their placement on the transplant waiting list. Over the past couple of years, however, UNOS has required transplant programs to send such a letter and keep documentation in their files as to when the letter was sent. But, patients should still check with their transplant team at their assigned hospital to find out if they have been placed on the national list. If you have questions about your status, your transplant coordinator will have all the answers for you.[5]

Close to 4,400 area men, women and children await life-saving organ transplants within the *Gift of Life* region serving the eastern half of Pennsylvania, southern New Jersey, and Delaware.

Local Waiting List (for that Pennsylvania, New Jersey, and Delaware region) as of March 1, 2004:
Kidney: 2,460
Heart: 127
Liver: 1,079
Kidney/pancreas: 220
Lung: 330
Pancreas: 173
Heart/lung: 8

?

Question:
What does a transplant coordinator do?

Answer:
The transplant coordinator is like a "go-between" person for the medical team and the potential recipient and recipient family. The coordinator keeps both sides informed as to each other's situations. For example, if a waiting recipient has an infection and is on antibiotics, that person is taken off the list while being medicated, then for another two weeks after finishing medication because he or she would not be able to have a transplant while sick. If the recipient family doesn't tell the transplant coordinator

this, and an organ comes up and the coordinator takes the time to track down your family member (which may take a few phone calls), then that precious time is wasted when it could have been used to reach the next person on the list.

Likewise, if the transplant coordinator calls a recipient family and tells that family to get to the hospital immediately because an organ is available, but then neglects to call them back to say, "Oh, never mind, there was an accident when retrieving the organ and it got sliced a bit, so it is useless now. Sorry for the false alarm," that would devastate a family, making it wary of the coordinator's abilities.

It is essential for the coordinator to have a close relationship with the recipient family, as well as the transplant team of doctors, nurses, social workers, and so forth. You need to have open communication with each other and stay in contact. (The posttransplant nurse will be a good contact person for you to keep in mind if any questions or problems ever come up, too.)

Eight years after his transplant, my dad is still in constant contact with Kathy Dasgupta, his posttransplant nurse at University of Chicago Hospital. Because she knows his history, he feels comfortable keeping her informed. He knows there won't be problems with his medical history if he forgets to mention certain details. There have been times when other nurses missed details on a chart and serious complications could have occurred if my dad didn't say something or ask a question.

? Question:
Can I be on "the list" at more than one hospital?

Answer:
Yes. UNOS policies permit "multiple listing." However, each hospital has its own criteria for listing patients and may have different rules about patients listing at other hospitals.[6]

? Question:
How many hospitals have transplant centers in the United States?

Answer:
According to the most current published data at UNOS, as of June 2003, there were 254 medical institutions in the United States operating an organ transplant program. This list will show

you just how many places there are per type of transplant. These transplant centers include the following active programs:

Type of Program	Number of Centers
Heart-Lung	73
Heart Transplant	139
Intestine	44
Kidney	245
Liver	123
Lung	70
Pancreas	138
Pancreas-Islet	37
TOTAL:	869

? **Question:**

Are transplant centers in every state? If not, which have them and how many centers are in each of those states?[7]

State	Numbers of Centers	State	Numbers of Centers
Alabama	1	Mississippi	1
Arizona	2	Missouri	6
Arkansas	3	Nebraska	3
California	16	New Jersey	2
Colorado	4	New Mexico	1
Connecticut	2	New York	9
Dist. of Columbia	4	North Carolina	5
Florida	8	Ohio	6
Georgia	3	Oklahoma	4
Hawaii	1	Oregon	2
Illinois	10	Pennsylvania	9
Indiana	3	Puerto Rico	1
Iowa	3	South Carolina	1
Kansas	2	Tennessee	5
Kentucky	3	Texas	14
Louisiana	4	Utah	4
Maryland	2	Virginia	7
Massachusetts	5	Washington	3
Michigan	5	Wisconsin	4
Minnesota	3		

Here is a great checklist to share with your parents of important questions to ask the hospital regarding money issues and insurance:

Insurance and money issues

◎ What is the average cost for a transplant, including care required before and after transplant?
◎ Will my insurance cover the transplant?
◎ Will my insurance require preapproval for any of my treatment?
◎ Should I get a second opinion from another doctor?
◎ Will I need to make a down payment or deposit? If so, approximately how much will it be?
◎ Will the insurance pay for my family and me to travel to a transplant center?
◎ Is there a waiting period on my insurance? If so, am I in a waiting period now?
◎ Will I have to pay for a portion of the costs? If so, approximately how much?
◎ Who will pay for my donor costs?
◎ Is there a dollar limit on my insurance for my transplant?
◎ Is there a time limit on my coverage?
◎ Are my medication costs covered by my insurance?
◎ Is there a time limit on the coverage for my medications?
◎ Who should I contact with questions concerning my insurance?
◎ Do any programs provide financial assistance for transplant patients?[8]

MINI-GLOSSARY, AT-A-GLANCE

The lists of terms will be alphabetized so you can just breeze through them quickly. This is only a sample of a much larger list of terms you will find at the Transplant Health website located at www.transplanthealth.com. The definitions are in the glossary, in the back of the book. (I have shortened or clarified some definitions for easier reading.

ABO typing

Accelerated rejection

Acute rejection

Adverse reaction

Allocation

Antibody

Antigens

Antirejection drugs

Chronic

Chronic rejection

Crossmatch

Delayed graft function

Donor

Edema

End-stage organ disease

Experimental treatment

Foreign body

Graft survival

Harvest

Hemorrhage

HLA system

Hyperacute rejection

Immunity

Nonfunction

Organ

Panel reactive antibody (PRA)

Recipient

Rejection

Retransplant

Status

Survival rates

Transplant center

UNOS

Waiting list

Xenotransplant

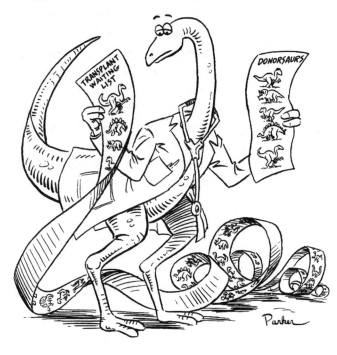

Gift of Hope Organ and Tissue Donor Network

The Gift of Hope Organ and Tissue Donor Network is the organ procurement organization (OPO) coordinating organ and tissue donation for Illinois and northwest Indiana, one of 59 such federally designated OPOs serving the United States. It has such a user-friendly website and an immeasurable amount of information, so no matter where you live in the country, you will find plenty of information helpful.

Of course, various organizations cover each of the 11 regions around the country and you can find them on the web by using whatever search engine you prefer, like Google.com, for example. But www.giftofhope.org is one of the best I have used, along with the United Network for Organ Sharing (UNOS).

Emergency Back-Up: **The UNOS Organ Center places many organs and also helps members with running computer matches, arranging transport for organs, updating patient records, and providing information about organ-sharing policies. The Organ Center is staffed 24 hours a day, 7 days a week, 365 days a year. If a catastrophe prevents use of the current facilities, operations can be switched in minutes to a fully equipped disaster recovery site.[9]**

United Network for Organ Sharing (UNOS)

Although the first successful kidney transplant was performed in 1954, the first simultaneous kidney/pancreas transplant performed in 1966, and the first successful liver transplant performed in 1967, it wasn't until 1968 (the same year the first successful isolated pancreas transplant and also the first successful heart transplant were performed) that the Southeast Organ Procurement Foundation (SEOPF) was formed as a membership and scientific organization for transplant professionals. In 1977, SEOPF implemented the first computer-based organ matching system, dubbed the "United Network for Organ Sharing" and that is how UNOS began.

All patients on waiting lists at various transplant centers are registered with UNOS. Its specialists run the national computer network that connects all the transplant centers and organ-donation organizations in the United States. UNOS is the organization that runs "the list."

Transplant Trivia: **In 1804, the first successful skin transplants between sheep and other animals reported.** **—G. Baronio, Milan.**[10]

The UNOS website (www.UNOS.org) is sure to be able to answer all your questions, if necessary. In fact, many other websites from various transplant organizations have a link to the UNOS website on their own site, so people who can't find the answers they are looking for can just click over to UNOS. It's like a "safe catch all" for any transplant information you would need. If you're feeling lost and overwhelmed, don't. You've made a huge step looking at this book and websites like the United Network for Organ Sharing will give you peace of mind, too.

If all else fails, because transplant information literally changes by the day, the Internet is the best place to search for cutting-edge updates on the latest procedures and laws.

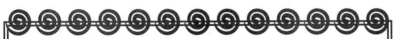

Here are a few great transplant websites I recommend, arranged alphabetically, not by any preference. After doing research for my family and then for this book, I visited these quite often. These sites will provide questions and answers you don't even know to ask. Plus they help explain the unbelievable amount of medical terms that will be thrown around a conversation.

www.americantransplant.org/transplant_glossary.htm
www.giftofhope.org
www.transplanthealth.com
www.unos.org
www.kidskare.org

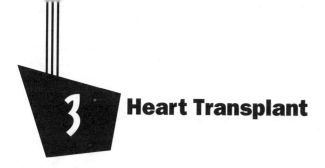

3 Heart Transplant

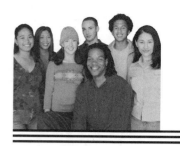

THE TECHNICAL STUFF: Q AND A

? Question:
What is a heart transplant?

Answer:
The medical term for a heart transplant is really cardiac transplantation. It means a surgical procedure that takes out a patient's diseased or injured heart and replaces it with a healthy, donor heart.

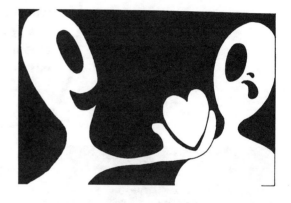

? Question:
Why is a heart transplant needed?

Answer:
Patients with end-stage heart failure or some other life-threatening heart disease need to have a heart transplant in order to survive. Not only will it save the person's life, it will improve the quality of life the person already has. Most patients who need a transplant are not well enough to lead a normal life. Some are hospitalized or have to at least quit working because they are so fatigued, tired, and have no energy. Replacing the patient's diseased heart with a healthy donor heart most often allows the recipient to go back to a regular life, such as work and day-to-day activities, and even allows a person to play sports in many cases.[1]

"Just walking from the refrigerator to a chair would make my dad winded," says Kevin, 16 years old. "But then it was cool because two months after his heart transplant, he could already run a mile!"

Kevin's sister Cheryl added, "I didn't notice his decline until after the surgery when we looked at photos from my graduation. He had very exaggerated circles under his eyes, plus his hair turned gray and a lot fell out during that time."

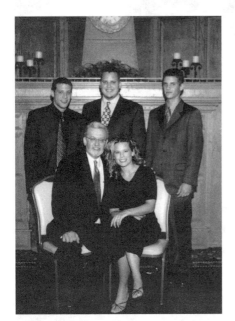

Dr. Dave Goodwin, heart recipient from cover photo, with children Cheryl, Robert, Mike, Kevin Goodwin.

? Question:

So why can't everyone with a "bad" heart be put on the transplant list?

Answer:

Because there are so many people with "bad" hearts, there has been a strict set of guidelines set up to make sure the people who really need a new heart to save their lives, not just improve the quality of life they already have, are able to get one first.

Here are some conditions that might cause a person to be excluded from the National Organ Transplant waiting list:[2]

Active infection

Pulmonary hypertension (high blood pressure)

Chronic lung disease with loss of more than 40% of lung function

Untreatable liver or kidney disease

Diabetes that has caused serious damage to vital organs

Disease of the blood vessels in the brain, such as a stroke

Serious disease of the arteries

Mental illness or any condition that would make a patient unable to take the necessary medicines on schedule

Continuing alcohol or drug abuse.

? Question:
Who would be a good candidate for the recipient waiting list?

"I had no worries about my dad's surgery because he showed no worries," said 16-year-old Kevin.

"He had such a positive attitude that it really helped the whole family feel at ease," added Kevin's sister Cheryl.

Answer:
Someone who has end-stage heart disease that threatens to kill him or her, even after medical treatments (such as open-heart surgery, bypass surgery, etc.) have failed to correct the heart's problem(s). Before a person can be put on the transplant waiting list, they have to go through a series of tests and a thorough medical exam. Some of the tests include blood tests, x-rays, and tests of heart, lung, and other organ function. The reason for these tests is to show if a patient will be healthy enough to survive the transplant surgery. As you can imagine, it is hardly a "routine operation."

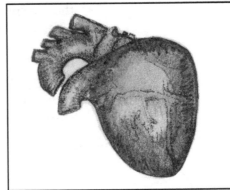

How long can a heart survive before being transplanted? A heart/lung transplant needs to happen within 4–6 hours from when the organ(s) is harvested from the donor. Heart valves and saphenous veins may be preserved from 3–10 years.[3]

Blood type is recorded because that is the first thing doctors look at when finding a compatible match. Also, a test called *PRA*, which stands for *panel reactive antibodies*, is done before a heart transplant is performed. The results show whether a patient is at high risk for something called a *hyperacute reaction*. That means a strong immune response against the new heart (which generally happens within minutes to hours after the new heart is transplanted).

If the PRA test shows the patient is high risk for this kind of reaction, then a cross-match is done between a patient and a donor heart before they will go ahead with transplant surgery. The cross-match will check how close the match is between the patient's tissue type and the donor heart tissue type. Because most people are not high risk and heart surgery is so immediate in nature, with the organ only surviving for 4–6 hours, a cross-match is usually not done.

?

Question:

Assuming my parent (for example) is well enough to be put on the transplant waiting list, what are the risks of surgery and what are the typical outcomes of these transplants?

Answer:

Any surgery poses risks, no matter if it is as simple as having your tonsils taken out or as complex as a heart transplant. The most common complications, and most dangerous, for transplant patients are organ rejection and infection. Most heart recipients have a rejection episode soon after transplantation, but doctors can usually diagnose it and respond immediately with treatment. They give a combination of immunosuppressive drugs in higher doses. That successfully treats the majority of the rejection cases.

Most infections are a side effect of the immunosuppressive drugs. It makes the person's immune

The outcome of a heart transplant depends on the patient's age, health, and various other factors. Approximately 73% of heart transplant patients are still alive 4 years after surgery.[4]

system unable to fight bacteria, viruses, and other microorganisms adequately. If a patient develops infections he or she may need to have the immunosuppressive drugs changed or perhaps just have the dose adjusted. It is difficult to fine-tune these things, but that's why such highly trained specialists take care of these problems.

Other complications that might happen right after surgery are:

Bleeding

Pressure on the heart, caused by fluid in the space surrounding the heart (this is also called pericardial tamponade)

Irregular heart beats

Reduced cardiac output

Increased amount of blood in the circulatory system, or

Decreased amount of blood in the circulatory system.[5]

?

Question:

Okay, my parent, my friend, or even I made it on "the list." Now what?

Answer:

A patient approved for a heart transplant is placed on the waiting list of a heart transplant center. (Not all transplant centers transplant every organ. While most do various transplants, many centers specialize in a certain organ. For example, some do heart/lung transplants, and others do a majority of liver transplants, etc.). All patients on waiting lists at various transplant centers are registered with UNOS, which organizes the waiting list for the entire country.

While waiting for a heart transplant, patients are given treatment to keep the heart as healthy as possible. They are checked regularly to make sure the heart is pumping enough blood. If it isn't, then intravenous medications may be used, and if those don't work, a mechanical pump can help keep the heart functioning until a donor heart becomes available.

?

Question:

There's a heart available, so who gets it?

"My friends knew something was up with my family . . . but my dad didn't tell me he was on the list almost until it was time to go in for the transplant. I didn't really talk about exact details with my friends."
—Kevin, 16 years old

Answer:

When a donor heart does become available, as much information as possible is entered into the UNOS computer. Different details are compared between the donor heart and patients on the waiting list. Patients are ranked according to blood type, body size and frame, size of the heart, how urgently the person needs a heart to live, and so forth. Because the heart and lungs are organs with the shortest amount of time to survive once retrieved from the donor, it is literally a race against the clock.

First the list of local patients who live within driving distance of the transplant center are checked for a good match. If none are found, the search goes out farther to a regional list. And if there still isn't a good enough match, the search is opened up to the national list to find the best matching recipient. The patient's transplant team of heart and transplant specialists makes the final decision to say whether the donor heart is really suitable for the patient. The patient has to be reachable; not have a cold, infection, or other illness; and be ready to get to the hospital immediately.

1967 = First successful heart transplant; 1981 = First successful heart-lung transplant.[6]

THE ACTUAL SURGERY

Okay, leaving the emotional part out of the equation (that is a whole mess in itself, so put it on the back burner for now), we'll go through what happens next. Say the heart becomes available and is approved for your parent (or you, or whoever needs the transplant). It is retrieved from the donor, packed in a sterile cold solution, and rushed to the hospital where the recipient is waiting. We'll walk through the eight basic steps to give you an overview of what will be happening:[7]

The anesthesiologist, who specializes in cardiovascular anesthesia, will give the patient medicine to essentially knock him or her out so he or she won't feel, hear, or remember the surgery.

Patients are often given antibiotics in their IV (*IV* stands for *intravenous line*, which is a bag and tube hooked up by a needle into the patient's hand or arm, that supplies medications directly into a vein) to prevent infections near the incisions and areas cut open during surgery.

The doctors use the cardiopulmonary bypass procedure (see Glossary) where a machine acts like the heart and lungs while the old and new organs are being exchanged.

After doctors are certain that enough blood is being circulated, the diseased heart is removed.

The new (donor) heart is attached to the patient's blood vessels.

Once the blood vessels are connected, the surgeons warm up the new heart and it begins beating. If the heart doesn't start to beat immediately, the surgeon might start it with an electrical shock.

The patient is taken off the bypass machine.

The patient is given medications to stimulate and maintain a regular heartbeat for the first 2 to 5 days after surgery. By then, the new heart should function normally by itself.

POSTSURGERY: Q AND A

?

Question:
Is the new heart really working now?

Answer:
As with all transplant recipients, the patient is given immunosuppressive drugs to prevent the body from rejecting the new organ. These drugs

Because the heart nerves are cut during a transplant operation, a transplanted heart usually beats a little faster than a recipient's original heart.[8]

31

are usually started before or during the heart transplant surgery. The immunosuppressive drugs keep the body's immune system from recognizing and attacking the new heart as foreign tissue. It allows the new heart to function properly like a natural part of the patient's body. The only problem for the patient is that with his or her immune system lowered, or compromised, it elevates his or her risk for more infections and other bad effects to happen.

Because rejection happens most often in the first few months after surgery, recipients usually get a combination of three or four immunosuppressive drugs in high doses in the beginning. After it has been established that the organ is working well and there are no signs of rejection, the drugs are lowered to maintenance doses. Recipients have to remain on these immunosuppressive drugs for the rest of their lives.

> "My parents were going through a divorce during the whole transplant waiting period, so it was awkward. . . . I was surprised by how my dad's muscles atrophied so quickly. There was a lot of stuff I still had to do for him after the surgery, too, that I hadn't expected."
> —Beth, 20 years old

? Question:
What happens right after surgery?

Answer:
Patients get taken to the ICU (intensive care unit) of the hospital so they can be carefully monitored, usually for the first 24–72 hours after surgery. A lot of these patients will need to be on oxygen for the first 4–24 hours following surgery. In the ICU, nurses and doctors will continue to monitor their patients' blood pressures, heart functions, and other organ functions carefully.

After the ICU, a patient's hospital stay varies. You'll see in the personal story below heart recipient Dr. Goodwin made it in and out in record time and returned to work within 30 days! Still others take a considerably longer amount of time. Do your best not to compare your family to other people's stories you've heard.

The chapter "Any Regrets?" contains a very personal story of what happens when jealousy creeps in. You can get caught up in feeling "why is that patient joking around with her kids while my dad is still whacked out on morphine, not even knowing who or where he is?" All jealousy does is hurt feelings and waste energy. Every single person has his or her own special timetable of what is needed to recover. There is no set rule, so if you or your parent takes a lot longer, or even much shorter, time to recover than is "average," don't sweat it.

? Question:

Are you sure I am (or my parent is) well enough to leave the hospital? I don't know how to do any nursing or medical stuff to help with aftercare!

Approximately 85% of patients return to work and other daily activities after receiving a new heart. Many are even able to participate in sports.[9]

Answer:

Don't worry. For the first 6 to 8 weeks after heart transplant surgery, patients usually come back to the transplant center twice a week for physical exams and medical tests. The tests will check for any signs of infection, rejection of the new heart, or any other complications.

Other tests might be done in addition to the other stuff done at the weekly visits. Some of the tests might include:

Five key terms you'll probably hear regarding a heart transplant (see Glossary in back for full definitions):

Cardiopulmonary bypass

Echocardiogram

End-stage heart failure

Endomyocardial biopsy

Immunosuppressive drug

Lab tests to check for infection

Chest x-rays to check for early signs of lung infection

> **Electrocardiogram (also called *ECG* or *EKG*) to check heart function by measuring the electrical activity of the heartbeat**
>
> **Echocardiogram (see Glossary) to check function of the ventricles in the heart**
>
> **Blood tests to check liver and kidney function (if these organs lose function, it could mean the heart is being rejected)**
>
> **CBC (complete blood counts) to check the numbers of blood cells**
>
> **Endomyocardial biopsy (see Glossary) to check for signs of rejection.**

? Question:

How will my family pay for it all?

Answer:

Depending on where the transplant takes place, if your family will need to travel or stay at hotels for a while and if there are any complications during or after surgery, the average cost for heart transplant surgery and the first year of follow-up care generally add up to around $250,000.

After the first year, daily medications and the medical tests that have to be done to maintain your parent's health will probably come to around $21,000 per year.

Hopefully, your parents have medical insurance. Different companies cover different amounts of transplant surgeries. Most commercial insurance companies pay a percentage of the costs, while Medicare will pay for the whole heart transplant if the surgery is performed at Medicare-approved centers. Medicaid will pay for heart transplants in 33 states and in the District of Columbia.[10] (If you haven't read Chapter 2 yet, which discusses "General Info to Know," turn back to it to review a great list of questions your parents and you should ask regarding costs and financing of a transplant.)

PERSONAL STORY: DR. DAVE GOODWIN— HEART RECIPIENT

While trying to get a job one summer at a Jewel Warehouse (Chicago land grocery chain), 19-year-old Dave Goodwin was put through an extremely thorough company physical. The job had extensive physical labor involved, so the company had strict rules about any health risks, no matter how small. While being examined, a heart murmur was detected, so the company stamped Dave unemployable and recommended he have it checked out.

Dave went to St. Luke's Hospital for an EKG (or echocardiogram) where it was discovered that there was an irregularity. He had an inverted T-wave, which led doctors to request further testing with an invasive heart catheterization. Since this was back in the 1970s and the procedure was much less commonly done, it involved a 1% risk of death to the patient. This test would not help correct any heart problem, only detect something wrong, so his mother said, "no thanks!" and that was the end of Dave's trip to the hospital.

Although he knew he had an enlarged heart, it really gave him no problems in his daily life, so he just went on with life as usual not thinking about his heart problem again. As Dave got older and finished school, he became an optometrist (eye care specialist), got married, and had four children. It wasn't until many years later, on a cold Chicago morning in January 1995, that a problem finally arose.

That morning, while getting ready for work, an odd thing happened. As his wife went downstairs to make lunches for the kids and have coffee, she decided to go back upstairs to get her new slippers, since the floor was cold. Usually, she wouldn't have returned upstairs until after her husband had finished showering, shaving, and getting ready for work. Then she'd go up and get dressed. But for some reason, that day she went back upstairs right away.

When she got there, she found her husband lying on the floor, foaming at the mouth, and he appeared to be choking. She yelled for their daughter Cheryl to call 911.

When the paramedics arrived they discovered Dave had a V-fib (or ventricular fibrillation), which means an irregular, extremely rapid heartbeat, which doesn't pump blood to the body or lungs. From the time the paramedics were called, got to the house, accessed the situation, and defibrillated Dave's heart, 8 minutes had passed. That is a dangerously long time for oxygen to be cutoff from the brain. Dave was resuscitated, but he was in a coma. His family was told that there was a good chance that he had suffered severe brain damage from the extended period without oxygen.

When Dave awoke from the coma, surprisingly he was coherent enough to ask where he was and what had happened. Then he asked why wasn't he at Loyola Hospital. This probably wasn't the best thing to ask the excellent staff at Edward Hospital, but they were happy to hear him ask a sincere question. (Dave's son had severe heart troubles in childhood and was helped tremendously by Loyola, so that's the heart facility Dave was familiar with.)

What's Your Name Again?

Although his initial alertness made his family happy, they quickly learned that he did suffer from short-term memory loss. For example, a friend would be visiting with him for a while, then leave briefly to go to the washroom and come back 5 minutes later only to have Dave say, "Hi! How have you been? It's so good to finally see you!" not realizing they had been talking for an hour already. Luckily, that problem corrected itself gradually after 2 to 3 days.

As if by miracle, doctors confirmed Dave had sustained zero brain damage and he was released and back to work in 2 weeks. He was referred to another hospital for follow-up (Northwestern—also in Chicago, due to a family connection). The good news, they told him, was that he had a defibrillator implanted in his chest, which would treat his arrhythmia if it occurred again. The bad news was that the 43-year-old doctor's condition would continue to worsen, and his heart probably wouldn't keep him alive past 50 years old. His wife and children were in shock and didn't quite know how to take the news. Dave was such an optimist that he tried to keep a positive attitude for himself and his family. He led by example.

Life Changing Experience: "My dad never seemed too religious before, but right before his [transplant] surgery, he started going to church. That was kind of a change from what we were used to. But it was obviously a life-changing experience, because years later, he still goes." —Cheryl, 25 years old

Every 3 months from then on, Dave had to undergo routine stress tests and work-ups at Northwestern. He wanted to be on the organ transplant list, but was told he wasn't sick enough. Since Northwestern was going through major changes, building a new center and was temporarily without a transplant unit, they referred Dave to Loyola, his original request when coming out of a coma.

Loyola routinely did heart catheterization tests to determine the pressure in Dave's heart along with heart function every 3 months. He also had an EKG, x-rays, and treadmill tests to see if he could reach a point where he had bad enough scores to be eligible for a transplant.

Doctors always commented on how Dave's attitude didn't match his test scores. According to the tests, he should have been severely fatigued and complaining about several things at once! In fact, the doctors joked they'd seen corpses with better numbers, although Dave continued to act fine.

Dave feels he was just so used to the gradual weakening and feeling awful that it simply felt normal to him. He didn't feel that complaining would be very productive, so he did his best to keep a positive attitude.

Because oftentimes a bad situation has something good come out of it, Dave's situation was no different. His stress test scores eventually got bad enough that he became a candidate for the national organ recipient waiting list. Although that sounds like really bad news, it was really very good because now he would have a chance to get a new, healthy heart.

After examining his support system, his ability to function at work, and overall health, he was added to the UNOS list in May 1995. In addition to his wife and kids, Dave was lucky to have six siblings who lived close by and were very helpful and supportive.

Your Support System

As a teen and young adult, you have things like exams, a boyfriend or girlfriend, a part-time job, college applications, and tons of other things that might have to be put on hold at a moment's notice, if possible. If you don't feel comfortable confiding in your parents (after all, how can you tell your parent, "I'm afraid you might die?" when you are supposed to help keep them calm and thinking positively?), try to find friends or perhaps even an older person you feel comfortable talking honestly with, like a former teacher or a counselor. It might even be easier to talk to strangers about such personal thoughts, so you could try a support group.

A great link to find a support group near you is www.transplanthealth. com/is/is_aso_sup.html. It shows the 11 transplant regions in the United States and will help you find the support group closest to you.

Plan Ahead as Much as Possible

Life is full of many stressors. Do yourself a favor and simplify as much as possible for now. If you have a backup plan to get things done if and when you need to put things on hold for a couple weeks, you'll be able to stay with your parents around the clock if you want.

If you have a part-time job, you should make your boss aware of your family's situation. Hopefully, if the manager is decent, he or she will be flexible enough to let you change hours when the time comes for your parent's surgery. You might want to talk to you coworker friends to see if they can be your backup if you need to call them. If you are the one waiting for a transplant, then I'm sure you really aren't too worried about some part-time job!

Another Step Backward

Only a few months after finally getting on the UNOS list, in early 1996, the criteria for those needing a heart transplant were reviewed and altered. So many people were on the list that the transplant committees made revisions to keep some people in treatment longer before attempting an actual transplant. Unfortunately, Dave fell under this category where they felt it was not a major threat to continue close medical monitoring and supervision. Therefore, he was taken off the UNOS list.

Being taken off was a frustrating blow to Dave. After years of quarterly testing and monitoring to finally get on the list, it was a scary situation that was out of his control. He had no voice or vote. As it is, solid organs such as hearts are in such huge demand and such short supply that many people are left to die waiting on the list. That's why the criteria had to be fine-tuned, to get the most urgent patients in line for the surgery.

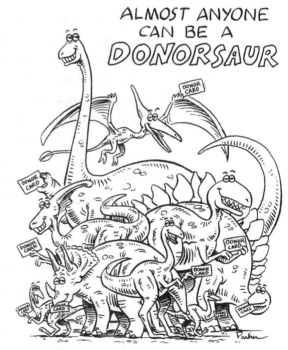

ALMOST ANYONE CAN BE A DONORSAUR

One major obstacle for Dave to get a transplant was that he was 6'2" and 195 pounds (a very large man to try and match up body and tissue types). He also has "O positive" blood ("O+"). "O positive" blood is a great type to have when you are a donor because anyone can use your blood, so the blood bank loves you. However, it's not so good if you need blood because only that specific type blood can help you. It really limits your available donors.

By January 2000, Dave was put back on the UNOS list because of a dramatic drop in his quarterly stress test scores of his heart rate function. Doctors even wanted him admitted to the hospital. Not only was he the sole income for his family of six, if he had to lay in a hospital bed watching the minutes tick by, he said that would drive him into an early grave! He was used to working 7 days a week, and he decided to continue to work that way until he got called to surgery.

As time went on and Dave got weaker, he did have to adapt and make adjustments. Some days he wouldn't even carry in his briefcase because the extra weight would make such an added strain that it would cut his energy in half for the day. He still went in for his routine tests every 3 months, as he had for 6 years! And Dave was still working 7 days a week, which amazed doctors.

The Call

On Monday, August 7, 2000 around 1:00 P.M., Dave got an "urgent call" at work. Because it was a phone call and not his pager, he assumed something bad had happened to one of his kids. When he quickly went to the phone, he was a bit confused to hear the voice of Dr. Barbara Pisani, one of the cardiologists on his transplant team. She said that they believed they had a heart for him. He said something like, "What? Now?" and she replied, "Well, yes, today." Dave walked back to his patient and simply said, "I have to go now. Excuse me," and left. He didn't stop home for a quick bag of clothes, toiletries, and so forth. He went straight to the hospital.

> Twenty-two-year-old Cheryl was glad her dad was able to make it to her college graduation. It was a stressful time, between her dad's failing health and her finishing school. The day she got home from college was the day her dad got "the call" and went in to have his heart transplant.

Amazingly, the surgery took a mere 4 hours, and Dave was out of intensive care in 12 hours (see cover photo taken with his four kids 12 hours after surgery, then again on p. 26). He was released and sent home only 9 days after his surgery! He was even back at work seeing patients within 1 month. This was a man who, while being prepped for surgery 1 month earlier, astonished doctors. The surgeon asked how he came in, from what hospital, assuming he was on life support because his heart was so badly damaged and in failure, only to discover that he had come in straight from work.

His positive attitude has been completely contagious and you can see how and why he fared so well in such a huge undertaking. I'm sure the doctors in the transplant community refer to him often when describing an ideal patient!

Update: What Is Dave Goodwin Doing Now?

Recently, Dr. Dave Goodwin retired from his job of many years as a Wal-Mart optometrist, to open his own private practice.

DONATING BLOOD IS A QUICK & EASY WAY TO SAVE LIVES!

- Just one donation can save up to three lives
- Donating takes less than one hour
- Your body replenishes the donated blood in only eight weeks.[11]

(Chapter notes: ch. 3, note 11—Source: Pamphlet, Life Source, March 2002)

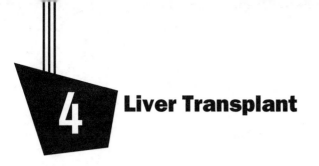

4 Liver Transplant

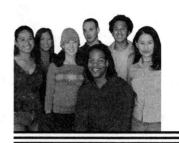

THE TECHNICAL STUFF: Q AND A

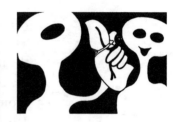

SIDEBAR 4.1: *WHAT ARE MELD AND PELD SCORES?*

Adults waiting for a liver transplant are assigned a MELD (Model for End-Stage Liver Disease) score. The score is based on the patient's risk of dying while waiting for a liver transplant, by evaluating a potential recipient's bilirubin, INR, and creatinine levels.

PELD (Pediatric End-Stage Liver Disease) is the score for candidates younger than 18 years old. The PELD score evaluates bilirubin, INR, and albumin levels along with growth failure and age when listed for transplantation. These help the transplant team predict how long a child has to live before getting a transplant.

The UNOS highly recommends patients review the MELD/PELD Q&A document on their website at www.UNOS.org, to help answer questions about the scores. They have a MELD/PELD calculator to help figure out your score, as well.[1]

Question:
What does your liver do?

Answer:
Your liver regulates energy so that you aren't too tired or too hyper; it keeps your energy level in check. It also makes proteins and keeps your blood clean, by removing waste.

? Question:

Why is a liver transplant needed?

Answer:

If your liver doesn't function properly, you will start having lots of problems with your health. Without your blood being cleaned, the toxicity will cause confusion, plus you'll have a hard time concentrating. Also, you could become very fatigued and unable to do routine things.

? Question:

Aren't live-donor liver transplants dangerous for the donor?

Answer:

The big controversy about a live-donor liver transplant involves the potential danger involved for the donor, even more than the recipient. The risk of death is lower than was originally thought; only three reported cases of donor death between 1993 and 2003, one of which was a suicide. However, the incidence of serious complications is a lot higher than expected.[2]

In December 2002, a report was completed addressing new guidelines on, among other things, informed consent and postoperative care of living donors.[3] The study was done to review adult liver donation in the state of New York for the New York State Council and the New York State Department of Health.

The American Liver Foundation really appreciated the report because the recommendations that come from the information will improve the quality of care and well-being of people who decide to be living donors. Improving the quality of life after a transplant is especially important for live-donors because that is when serious complications usually occur.

? Question:

What is Alpha 1-Antitrypsin deficiency?

Answer:

Alpha-1 Antitrypsin deficiency, also referred to as Alpha-1 or AAT deficiency, is one of the most common serious hereditary

SCANDAL

In July 2003, three Chicago hospitals were accused of skewing their liver transplant waiting lists as far back as 1995.

Although reports said there was no evidence that anyone had died for lack of transplant because some patients were moved up the list, some doctors said they felt it was quite possible someone could have. The reason a hospital might make people appear sicker than they really are, to get their transplants done quicker, is that there is a requirement for hospitals to perform 12 transplants a year for 2 years with a 75% or better survival rate in order to get reimbursed for the cost of the surgeries from Medicare and Medicaid.[4]

disorders in the world and can result in life-threatening liver or lung disease in children and adults. It often leads to hepatitis and cirrhosis. Rarely it causes a skin condition called *panniculitis*. It can also lead to lung destruction and is often misdiagnosed as asthma or smoking-related chronic obstructive pulmonary disease (COPD).

Lung disease is the most frequent cause of disability and early death among affected Alpha-1 persons, striking in the prime of life, and is a major reason for lung transplants. Alpha-1 can also lead to liver failure in childhood, making it a major cause of liver transplantation in children. It may also cause progressive liver damage in adults, often going undetected until reaching a critical, life-threatening stage.[5]

PERSONAL STORY: JOSH THOMPSON— LIVER RECIPIENT

Beating the odds with Alpha-1 is 13-year-old Josh Thompson of Orlando, Florida. Josh[6] was born with Alpha-1 Antitrypsin deficiency and the doctors who treated him in the early stages believed his chances for a long life were quite low.

When he was 3 months old, the doctor at Josh's regular checkup noticed he was a bit jaundiced. Mrs. Thompson said she thought so, too, but after having Josh checked out by a doctor on the military base where they lived, she was told not to worry about it.

Josh's new pediatrician did worry about it. In fact, he admitted Josh to the hospital for further tests and a liver biopsy. The biopsy (where a doctor takes out a small sample of the liver to examine it) showed a bunch of scarring for such a young infant. His parents, Tish and John, were really surprised by the news because there was no history of liver disease on either side of their families. They had never even heard of Alpha-1 disease!

The Thompsons were told Josh's life expectancy was low, according to the doctor who did the biopsy. Yet Josh continued to thrive and surprised them all. He stayed healthy throughout his early childhood. His mom said, "Josh seemed to be completely normal, except for elevated liver enzymes. He went from monthly checkups to going only once a year."

It wasn't until he was 10–years old that real health problems started. In addition to his enzymes still climbing, his spleen (another organ) was greatly enlarged. Doctors told Josh's parents that their son would eventually need a liver transplant. Tish and John heard great things about a transplant center in Pittsburgh, so they went there to get their son evaluated. His name was put on the UNOS waiting list after they met with the transplant team.

In 1967 the first successful liver transplant was performed.[7]

Over the next year, Josh had frequent fevers and infections and his health kept getting worse, but still no liver arrived. The family decided to return to Florida to explore other options. They searched around again and learned of a center in Miami, Florida, that did a lot of transplants. They made an appointment to meet with the people at that center. Not only was the location more convenient, being in the same state and closer to home, but they also had hopes for a much shorter waiting list.

Luckily, 3 days after being evaluated, a liver became available and the whole family flew to Miami immediately. Josh had his surgery on February 25, 1995, and made it home on March 20 to celebrate his parents' wedding anniversary. "It was the best gift we could have imagined," said Tish Thompson.

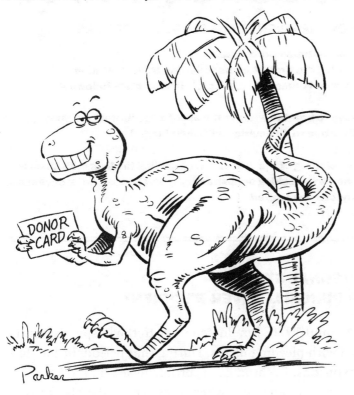

DONORSAURS
GIVE LIFE A SECOND CHANCE

DONOR CARD

Parker

Never as Bad as You Think

According to his mother, Josh said, "The surgery wasn't nearly as bad as I had expected." She said he's a regular eighth grader, quite social, who takes his anti-rejection medicine without any problems or reactions. So far, he has had no ill effects from the transplant.

Josh just wants to be treated like a normal kid, which is just what his parents do. Tish said, "We don't talk about the transplant much anymore. We've moved beyond it."

When asked about the donor family, Tish says she wrote them a letter of appreciation. "There was no way I could really thank them. That was the hardest letter I ever had to write," she said. "Just think about it: for my child to live, some else's child had to die." They learned later that the donor was a 3-year-old child who had died in a car accident.

SEVEN KEY HURDLES OF THE LIVER TRANSPLANT PROCEDURE

- Surviving the liver transplantation procedure.
- Bleeding (internally) during the first 24 hours following transplantation.
- Determining if the new liver is functioning properly immediately following transplantation.
- Becoming strong enough to breathe without the aid of a respiratory machine. (Liver patients are especially prone to difficulties with their lungs.)
- Infection.
- Technical problems (i.e., clotting of the vein or artery feeding the liver = 3% chance; the bile duct from the new liver leaking or obstructing = 8% chance.) *Note: Uncommon problems, if found early, can be repaired.*
- Rejection.[8]

PERSONAL STORY:
JIM PURCELL—LIVER RECIPIENT

Around 1970, Jim Purcell went to the hospital several times with bleeding ulcers. During that period, he had blood transfusions. Eventually, his problems led him to have a gastric resection (where they removed 60% of his stomach). It is almost certain that one of the transfusions he received was blood from an individual who had Hepatitis C.

Approximately 15–18 years later, Jim became ill with what he felt was the flu. However, because it seemed to go on way too long, he consulted with his doctor. Dr. Bob Trausch determined that Jim had cirrhosis of the liver.

In the United States in the 1980s the incidence of Hepatitis C was approximately 240,000 newly diagnosed people annually. By 1998, those figures dropped drastically to 40,000 new infections reported each year because of screening of donated blood according to the Centers for Disease Control.[9]

Facing Prejudice

The cirrhosis diagnosis came as a complete shock to Jim because he, like many others, thought that only people who were in the late stages of alcoholism had it. In fact, when telling people of his condition, they all looked at him differently and made ignorant comments like, "I didn't know you were such a big drinker!" assuming that he had inflicted this disease upon himself.

> *Defending Dad:* "It is weird, but I felt defensive for him [my father.] When I would tell people my dad needed a new liver, I'd always be quick to say that he had a tainted blood transfusion years ago and *that's* why he was sick." —Tina, early 20s

Jim started seeing a gastroenterologist who worked at Rush-Presbyterian-St. Luke's Hospital in Chicago. He continued with that doctor for 5 or 6 years. One day, he felt like he was filling up with water. When he went in to the doctor's office, a procedure was done that punctured his stomach with needles and almost a gallon of fluid was drained out! He lost 25 pounds immediately, then was put on a special diet and diuretics and lost an additional 15 pounds. After that episode, he was able to maintain his health steadily. Jim went along for another few years until at age 63 his health declined again and he was finally put on "the list." He felt he was finally on his way to recovering.

> After learning he had cirrhosis of the liver "I was devastated for several weeks. I assumed cirrhosis was what people in the gutter, close to death, had," said Jim, a liver recipient who contracted Hepatitis C from a blood transfusion during an abdominal surgery years earlier.

During his wait time, Jim felt that the most difficult symptom of his liver disease was having a bad memory, which made his decision making very difficult. Severe itching was another irritating side effect. He often got frustrated when trying to drive to well-known places like his son's house, or Soldier's Field (where the Chicago Bears football team plays) and even the airport, which he'd been to hundreds of times. It was especially upsetting to him to hear snide comments his younger kids made.

I didn't even remember this until my dad reminded me, but when he looped around past Soldier Field a third time, I guess I looked at my brother, rolled my eyes and said, "See what it's like with him?" I felt horrible that my dad remembers me saying that, and I told him I was sorry and ashamed. Although it will be hard for you, try to remember that whoever is sick needs your patience and compassion.

After making one final check of the insurance coverage, Jim was told, "A transplant will not be covered." He was shocked! He had checked on this coverage several times over the years to be sure a transplant would be covered and was repeatedly told, "Yes, it was fine." Now, his company said, "You were covered for treatment, but not for the actual surgery."

How long can a liver survive before being transplanted? A liver has up to 24 hours before deterioration begins and it is considered unusable.[10]

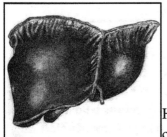

Jim was devastated with the news and felt all was lost. He and his family would have to come up with a huge chunk of money to somehow pay for the surgery. Amazingly, he was able to get back on his company's HMO insurance before it lapsed (since his wife's plan rejected him), but was told he had to go to the doctors at University of Chicago. Although this was an adjustment, because he had a long relationship with the other staff, Jim quickly learned that his new doctor, Dr. Alfred Baker, was considered the best liver specialist in North America. Jim felt he was with the best all-around team.

To top off his good news, being with an HMO now meant that the surgery would be covered 100% instead of just 80%. Because the bill for the surgery came to over $500,000, Jim and his family would have had to pay $100,000 out of their own pocket if he had not changed insurance companies. The HMO monitored his progress for over a year and its staff was full of people who were genuinely concerned.

As a young adult, insurance problems are probably not what you ever think about, but they are huge stressors for your parents. Just keep in mind that they need your emotional support to get through the entire ordeal, even if you're not sure what they're so frazzled about sometimes.

A SPOUSE SPEAKS OUT

As a wife of a liver recipient and the mother of five worried children I wondered if people knew what the family goes through. I had wished that I had a group to talk to, a therapist who understood the changes in behavior of all those involved, or a book. My daughter, the author of the book you are reading, decided to write one when she felt the same frustrations from lack of information (especially just emotional "heads up") for family members. It's not easy to talk about fears and frustrations and go through those feelings again and again, but I'm glad she did.

The fact is, it is scary to watch your loved one's personality change as his/her disease progresses, and there is nothing you can do about it. I can say, in my husband's case, the fogginess disappeared after a few weeks following surgery, his anger has lessened, and preoccupation with the whole process, which was high at first, has faded, allowing for life to return to normal again.

I wish you hope, patience, and love, whether you have been through a long and tedious journey or are just beginning it. May it end happily for each and every one of you as it has for my family. (P.S. Remember, attitude is key!) —Diane Purcell, wife of liver recipient

"How long will I wait?" Jim questioned. The doctors estimated that he would be on the UNOS list for maybe a year or so. It turned out he waited just over 9 months. He was very fortunate. When asked if he would have considered any of his family members to be "Live Liver Donors" to him, he said, "No. I wouldn't want them to jeopardize their health for me at age 63."

Shortly before his daughter's wedding (mine) in 1995, Jim was hospitalized and was moved up to 25th on the liver waiting list. He was given a pager and told the wait would probably be around 6 weeks. (You can see a photo of Jim, my dad, walking me down the wedding aisle in Chapter 7. Although it doesn't show in the photo, he was wearing his pager at the time!)

While waiting for the call to come, Jim's biggest concern with having a transplant was the period after the operation. When he remembered the surgery for his gastric resection, he knew that the first 2 weeks of recovery would be horrible and he dreaded that. He didn't give much thought to rehabilitation. He just figured in a few months he would be fine.

When asked if age was a factor, Jim was told there was not an official cut-off age because that would be age discrimination, but that he probably wouldn't get one after he was 65 years old, if it took that long.

As it turned out, he waited 16 weeks for his transplant. "The call" finally came in the fall during a Chicago Bears and Green Bay Packers football game. Because the teams are rivals, the game is always sold-out, and the traffic was sure to be a disaster! Luckily, the game was held in Wisconsin. Jim's transplant team wanted him downtown at the hospital in 2 hours or less. To travel from the northern suburbs to the south side of Chicago could have easily taken 2 hours with traffic, even if he left that very minute. Luckily, it was a beautiful, crisp day with light traffic.

"The hardest part while waiting for my aunt to get a liver transplant was to watch her confusion. It was hard to have faith that it would go away after the transplant and that she would return to her normal self," [with regular mental capabilities]. —Hannah, 21 years old

When he couldn't reach anyone in his entire family (wife and five kids, three of whom lived locally) and after tryng to reach friends in the neighborhood, without success, he started to panic. Jim's last resort was to call some friends, the Ramsays. He hated to do that because Bill Ramsay was quite ill and had less than a year to live. Because he was desperate, he did call Bill and Ann, who came immediately and drove him downtown.

Miraculously, they got there in record time with very little traffic. Jim wanted to see his wife, Diane (my mother), and his kids, but my mom and I were the only ones who arrived in time to see him before surgery, and essentially say good-bye just in case.

Because of staff error, one of my sisters was at the hospital after all, but was sent to the wrong room and told to wait there. By the time someone got her to the correct place, our father was already on his way to surgery. She didn't get to see him one last time.

"I was convinced that I would survive since Dr. Baker often said survival for patients healthy enough to come in of their own accord (as opposed to those brought by ambulance or who were already hospitalized) had approximately a 98% survival rate. I was confident, but still wanted to see Diane and the kids just in case," Jim said.

Of the surgery and the first memories after it, Jim recalls, "I remember conversations of the doctors, and the recovery in intensive care seemed to go on forever with a great deal of discomfort. I imagined a lot of things, like thinking the ceiling was a wall and that the hospital room was an annex of our home in Deerfield.

The TV was on and the football field looked like it was bent in the shape of a dogleg, like on a golf course instead of a normal rectangle. Mostly I remember how good it was to see the family there, waiting for me, but being so miserable with so many tubes attached to me."

Regarding the weeks following surgery, Jim said, "People always say you feel a little better each day, but I never noticed except for a week at a time. Fatigue and lack of strength were hard to overcome. My recovery from this surgery was even worse than I had feared it would be. Another thing I remember was breaking down a lot and crying often. Usually I'd cry when someone was especially nice; it just overwhelmed me."

Six weeks after his transplant surgery, Jim returned to work. He was upset to find he had lost his title as vice president of finance and would become assistant controller. His pay wasn't cut, but the job was a demotion. He insisted on negotiating a different title and they agreed upon "treasurer" but he felt, for the most part, his career was over. He felt ignored and kept out of decision making, then finally decided to retire in 1999. Right after he left the company (where he had worked for over 20 years), the sales dropped significantly.

"While it was a comfort for my dad to be able to return to work, the fact that he felt so disrespected after working there [at his previous company] my whole lifetime, was horrible to see," said Jim's daughter.
—Tina, early 20s.

Today, Jim feels good. He has some other health problems now as an aftermath of his illness and surgery, including high blood pressure, diabetes, and other smaller symptoms, but for the most part, he feels great. He is definitely happy to have made the decision to have the transplant because he would have died years ago without it.

Since his surgery, he has seen seven more grandchildren born into his family. He has retired to a house on a golf course, not far from some of his kids, and other than remembering to take his various medications, his daily life is not affected. He has moved past the surgery and doesn't really think about it much any more.

Hepatitis C Treatment: Side effects for treatment of Hepatitis C vary from mild to severe with symptoms ranging from fatigue, depression, thyroid problems, head and backaches, anemia, and hair loss. However, within weeks of treatment ending, symptoms subside. Several of those interviewed commented that the biggest help is having a support group of peers who have also survived Hepatitis C, who can empathize with what they are going through. Sometimes having someone going through the same thing at the same time can validate a person's feelings.

Four to five million Americans are infected with the Hepatitis C virus. Again, the amount of misinformation available on the World Wide Web came up. It was mentioned earlier by another teen that you couldn't have blind faith in Internet communities. Just because there is a website saying certain information, doesn't mean it has to be true or accurate. Make sure your sources are reputable, if you are taking the information to be fact.

PERSONAL STORY: STONEY WEISZMANN— DAUGHTER OF LIVER RECIPIENT

Stoney Weiszmann, whose parents have been married 50 years, and who has three sisters, was 32 years old when her father, George, had a liver transplant. The reason he needed a transplant was for a diagnosis of "hepatitis unknown." Doctors still are unclear how or when he contracted the disease.

At first Stoney was shocked and scared, but not totally surprised. When she and her sisters got a chance to meet with the surgeon to ask questions, it was a great comfort.

In hindsight, when asked if she would have done anything differently throughout this whole ordeal, Stoney commented, "I would have changed the total involvement that I was in. I am a control freak and I needed to be there and involved with everything. Later, that proved to be a mistake because I got sick and ended up in the emergency room of the hospital myself with massive stomach pains." She was told her stress level was out of control.

One of Stoney's biggest emotional obstacles was when her dad made everyone in the family come together to plan his funeral "just in case." It was something that calmed her dad's fears of getting everything in order, but was extremely difficult to deal with as a family member.

"Every time the phone rang I thought it could be the hospital," Stoney said. "I was afraid of him not making it through the surgery and was also nervous about the difficult recovery that would be coming too."

George Weiszmann ended up waiting on the list for a year–and–a half. Luckily, insurance did not prove to be a hassle, and out-of-pocket expenses were minimal. In fact, he was called to surgery days before his pager arrived. He went to the hospital immediately and Stoney and her sisters arrived an hour later. They were able to see him before he got wheeled into the operating room. It was a comfort for the whole family to be together once more and pray with George.

The surgery took 11 hours, and no major problems occurred. One potentially bad finding was the doctor found cancer in George's liver, but because it was so contained, it did not become an issue. His recovery time was very quick. The family was originally told to expect George to be in the hospital for probably a week, but by day four, he was ready to go home. On day seven after surgery, he developed an infection in his blood and was only given a 20% chance to live! He was put on a respirator and was unconscious for almost a week. Although doctors did not expect him to live, he was able to prove them all wrong and survived his serious setback.

Friends Are Great, but Can't Always Understand

Stoney's friends have been as supportive as they could be, but not having gone through the same ordeal, they didn't really understand what she was going through. Stoney wasn't even completely sure what she was going through with the whole traumatic event! You might be feeling that way, too.

One thing that helped Stoney was her involvement with the group Transplant Recipient International Organization (TRIO), mentioned in Chapter 8. (www.trio.org). Out of her group of approximately 20 people, she was the only nonrecipient. But she developed a good group of friends. She went to a conference for support members and caregivers and got to vent and cry and had people share their stories with her.

Today, George Weiszmann is alive and well, and his liver is functioning perfectly. "We thank God and the donor family for that every day," Stoney said. As for advice she could give others she said, "I guess I can say have faith and it will happen. Try to stay busy and get all the information you can get. Don't be afraid to ask the doctors questions. There are support groups that you can get involved in through the hospital or through the American Transplant Association. Talk to as many people as you can!"

A NEW CENTER FOR LIVER CANCER

Dr. Ronald W. Busuttil is head of the nation's busiest liver transplant program at UCLA. In 1992, he was the first surgeon to ever perform a split-liver transplant, where a donated liver is split in two and each piece is given to two different recipients. Now, thanks to a $2 million donation from the Dumont Foundation, a new center will be opening as a combined effort with UCLA's Jonsson Comprehensive Cancer Center.

The new center is called the Dumont–UCLA Liver Cancer Center. The reason to create a center that focuses solely on liver cancer is due to the inadequate efforts made to eliminate the disease.

Dr. Busuttil gathered the best scientists, physicians, surgeons, oncologists, liver specialists, and interventional radiologists. The hope is to study liver cancer to discover its causes and possible *cures*. In 2002, a million people died of the deadly disease in the United States.[11]

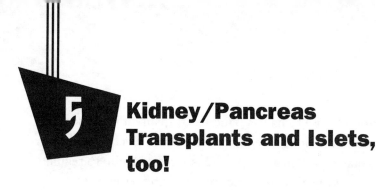

5 Kidney/Pancreas Transplants and Islets, too!

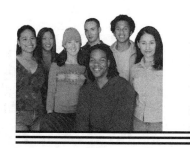

THE TECHNICAL STUFF: Q AND A

? Question:
What is a kidney/pancreas transplant?

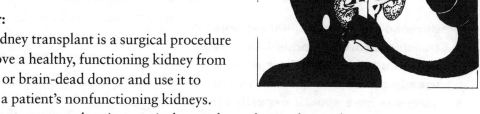

Answer:
A kidney transplant is a surgical procedure to remove a healthy, functioning kidney from a living or brain-dead donor and use it to replace a patient's nonfunctioning kidneys.

A pancreas transplant is a surgical procedure where a diseased pancreas is replaced with a healthy one from a compatible donor (after his or her death).

A kidney/pancreas transplant removes all three diseased organs (pancreas and two kidneys) and replaces them with two working organs (one kidney and one pancreas).[1]

> **Pancreatitis is an inflammatory condition of the pancreas that is painful and at times deadly.**

? Question:
Why is a kidney/pancreas transplant needed?

Answer:
When people have chronic kidney failure, or end-stage renal disease (see sidebar), they need either functioning kidneys (via transplant), or to be on dialysis permanently. Otherwise, their blood will not be properly cleaned of waste, and proper levels of certain kidney-regulated chemicals cannot be maintained, causing those people to die.

People choose to have a pancreas transplant because their pancreas can no longer regulate the glucose levels, which can lead to diabetes. A healthy pancreas secrets insulin to regulate glucose; a nonhealthy one does not, causing patients to dependent on giving themselves insulin every day to survive.[2]

Question:
Why can't everyone with a "bad" kidney and/or pancreas be put on the transplant list?

Answer:
Patients with a history of heart disease, lung disease, cancer, or hepatitis may not be suitable candidates for a kidney transplant. Many people with diabetes are not good candidates for a pancreas transplant alone. If they are successfully controlling their diabetes with insulin injections, then they are usually not considered for pancreas transplants.

Pancreas transplantation is major surgery that requires suppression of the immune system with immunosuppressive drugs, which have serious side effects. In 1996, 85% of pancreas transplants were performed simultaneously with kidney transplants, 10% were performed after a kidney transplant, and only 5% were performed as a pancreas transplant alone.[3]

Because only about 1,000 pancreas transplants are performed each year in the United States, the operation usually occurs at a hospital where surgeons have special expertise in the procedure.

Question:
Why do surgeons do kidney and pancreas transplants together?

Answer:
The big decision to get a pancreas transplant only (without a kidney transplant) depends on whether patients feel it is worth it to go through lifelong immunosuppressive drug treatments just to avoid lifelong insulin dependence. They would simply be exchanging one drug treatment for another.

The idea to transplant both organs at the same time was started when doctors thought that patients receiving immunosuppressive treatments for the kidney transplant might as well receive the benefit of a pancreas transplant as well.

TRANSPLANT TRIVIA

1954—First successful human kidney transplant between identical twins (Drs. Joseph E. Murray, John Hartwell Harrison and John P. Merrill performed the surgery at the Brigham Hospital in Boston, Massachusetts).
1959—First successful transplant of kidney between genetically different siblings (performed by Dr. Joseph Murray).
1962—First successful cadaver kidney transplant (performed by Dr. David Milford Hume).
1966—First successful kidney/pancreas transplant.
1988—First successful pancreas transplant (without transplanting kidney at same time).[4]

? Question:

Who would be a good candidate for the pancreas recipient waiting list?

Answer:

- Someone between ages of 20–40 years old
- People who have extreme difficulty regulating their glucose levels
- Those who have few secondary complications of diabetes
- Those who are in good cardiovascular (heart) health.

The pancreas is a small organ, approximately 6 inches long, located in the upper abdomen, connected to the small intestine. Its function is essential to the digestive process. The pancreas produces enzymes that help digest protein, fat, and carbohydrates before they can be absorbed through the intestine. Then it makes islands of endocrine cells that

THE PANCREAS AND SURROUNDING PARTS

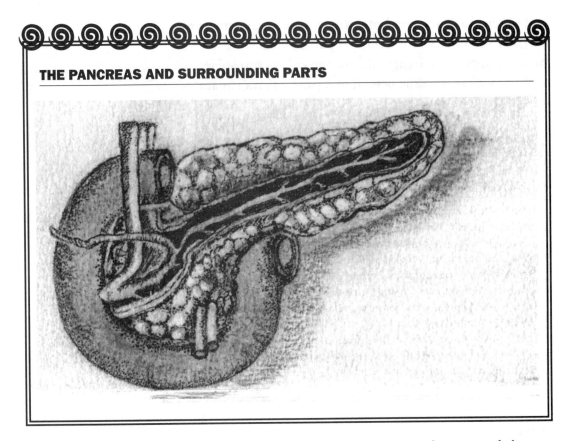

produce insulin, which controls the use and storage of glucose (sugar), which is the body's main energy source.

? Question:
What are Islets?

Answer:
In the pancreas, which is located behind the lower part of the stomach, insulin and enzymes are made to help the body use and digest food. Clusters of cells, called the *Islets of Langerhans*, are spread all over the pancreas. Islets are made up of two types of cells: alpha cells, which make a hormone called *glucagons* that raises the level of sugar in the blood, and beta cells, which make insulin.[5] Insulin helps the body use glucose for energy. If your beta cells don't produce enough insulin, diabetes will develop.

? Question:
What is an Islet transplant?

Answer:

Islet cell transplants began in 1974 as another way to possibly treat patients with diabetes. The hope is to help prevent organ damage associated with diabetes by allowing patients to receive the transplant in the earlier stages of their disease.

In a pancreatic Islet transplant, cells are taken from a donor pancreas (after the donor has died) and transferred into another person. Once implanted into the recipient, the new Islets begin to make and release insulin. The purpose is to help people with Type 1 diabetes live without daily injections of insulin. A great advantage of the procedure is that the cells are injected into a recipient with a needle, so it does not require general anesthesia or major surgery, and patients often go home the same day.

Because it is still in the early stages, these transplants are not done routinely yet. As with any transplant, rejection is the biggest problem, plus some patients who have received an Islet cell transplant have not had complete success. Some still require insulin to control their diabetes.

Recipients still have to take all the immunosuppressant drugs as any other transplant patient, and researchers do not fully know what long-term effects these drugs may have. Although test trials are very encouraging so far, more research is needed to answer questions about how long the Islets will survive and how often the transplantation procedure will be successful. Since it is considered investigational, many hospitals do not perform the procedure. Currently, only 34 U.S. hospitals perform Islet cell transplants according to UNOS.[6]

According to UNOS statistics, as of February 27, 2004, 330 patients were already on the waiting list for an Islet transplant. In the future, Islet cell transplantation may become the number one choice for treatment of diabetes, but for now, there are many other options for treating the disease.

? **Question:**

Who might be a good candidate for an Islet transplant?

Answer:

- ◎ **Persons between the ages of 18 and 65 years old**
- ◎ **Have had Type 1 diabetes for at least 5 years**
- ◎ **Unable to control blood sugar even with intensive therapy**
- ◎ **Unable to adequately sense the onset of hypoglycemia (low blood sugar)**
- ◎ **Have had at least one hypoglycemic reaction in the past 1.6 years that cannot be otherwise explained and required medical attention**
- ◎ **Have diabetes complications—such as blurred vision or kidney, nerve, or blood vessel problems—despite efforts to control blood sugar.**[7]

Question:
Assuming I am (or my parent is, for example) well enough to be put on the transplant waiting list, what are the risks of surgery and what are typical outcomes of these transplants?

Answer:

? As with all transplant surgery, the top three risks for pancreas transplantation are generally organ rejection, excessive bleeding, and infection. Diabetes and poor kidney function greatly increase the risk of complications from anesthesia during surgery.

The kidney transplant procedure carries risks for both a living donor and recipients. Excessive bleeding and infection are possible risks, as well as a urine leak, for kidney patients. In approximately 5% of kidney transplants, the ureter suffers some damage, resulting in a leak. But this problem is usually correctable with follow-up surgery.

A risk for both kidney and pancreas transplantation is the immunosuppressive medication that must be taken for the rest of the recipient's life. Because these drugs suppress (or slow down) the immune system, it is much easier for the patient to get infections. Plus these drugs can cause other bad side effects from high blood pressure to osteoporosis. (Side effects can be lessened with prescription and dosage adjustments, but are still possible dangers.)[8]

? Question:

Okay, I made it on "the list" (or my parent made it on the list.) Now what?

Answer:

Whoever is waiting for transplantation will be put through a complete study of blood and tissues to look for the closest compatibility with a perspective donor. You (or your parent) will also be given tests to see if you are healthy enough, mentally and physically, to withstand the actual procedure, and more importantly, the aftercare that will be required to stay alive.

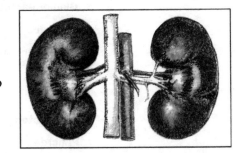

Donors (for kidney transplantation) undergo a complete medical history and physical exam to see if they are suitable for donation. Blood samples and tissue typing for antigen matches are studied to see if they are compatible with a potential recipient.

? Question:

There is a kidney and a pancreas available, so who gets them?

Answer:

After it is determined that a potential recipient is as closely matched to donated organs as possible, UNOS looks at how long the recipient has been on the list, and how urgent the surgery is for his or her survival (plus how much longer he or she can live without a transplant).

Also, the potential recipient must be within a certain distance from the transplant center, due to the timeliness of transplanting the organs while those organs are functioning properly after being removed from the donor.

How long can a pancreas and kidney survive before being transplanted? A pancreas can survive 12–24 hours; a kidney can survive 24–72 hours.[9]

MINI-GLOSSARY LIST OF TERMS (SEE GLOSSARY FOR DEFINITIONS):

BUN

Creatinine

Diabetes

Dialysis

Duodenum

ESRD

Glomerular filtration rate

Glucagon

Graft pancreatitis

Incision

Kidneys

Nephrectomy

Pancreas

Reflux nephropathy

Reflux pancreatitis

Rejection

Ureter

THE ACTUAL SURGERY

Once removed, kidneys from live donors and cadavers are placed on ice and flushed with a cold preservative solution. The kidney can be preserved in this solution for 24–48 hours until the transplant takes place. The sooner the transplant happens after harvesting the kidney, the better the chances are for it to still function properly.[10]

POSTSURGERY Q AND A

?

Question:

What happens right after surgery?

Answer:

Pancreas transplant patients are monitored closely for organ rejection. All vital body functions are watched closely as well.

The average hospital stay is 3 weeks, but it can take about 6 months to recover from surgery. Plus, recipients will take immunosuppressive drugs for the rest of their lives.

✳Kidney donors and recipients will experience some soreness where the incisions were made. Numbness, caused by severed nerves, near the incision may be experienced, too. A kidney recipient will have to take immunosuppressant drugs as long as that person still has the new kidney. Recipients may need to adjust their dietary habits because of side effects from the medications they are on (including increased appetite or sodium and protein retention).

?

Question:
Are you sure I am (or my parent is) well enough to leave the hospital? I don't know how to take care of myself (or my parent) after such a medical ordeal!

Answer:
In a successful transplant, the pancreas begins producing insulin and brings the regulation of glucose back under normal body control. This availability of insulin prevents additional damage to the kidneys and blindness associated with diabetes. Many patients report an improved quality of life.

With a new kidney, it may start working right away, but it may take several weeks to begin producing urine. This doesn't mean they won't start working eventually. It might just take some time. ✳Living donor kidneys are more likely to begin functioning earlier than cadaver kidneys because the cadaver kidneys were preserved and stored longer.

Patients may have to undergo dialysis for several weeks while their new kidney establishes an acceptable level of functioning. No matter whether it be a kidney, pancreas, or kidney/pancreas transplant, recipients will need to see their doctor at least twice a week during the first few months, on average, to monitor the transplant and check for signs of rejection.

✳Studies have shown that after they recover from surgery, kidney donors typically have no long-term complications from the loss of one kidney, and their remaining kidney will increase its functioning to compensate for the loss of the other.

? Question:

How will my family pay for it all?

Answer:

Chapter 2, "General Info to Know," contains a great checklist of financial questions. Refer to that section now.

PERSONAL STORY: CRYSTAL CAPSER—KIDNEY/PANCREAS RECIPIENT (TYPE I DIABETES—JUVENILE DIABETES)

Bad News Delivered

Crystal Capser remembers one specific visit to her doctor regarding her diabetes. Having dealt with the disease for 27 and a half years, since childhood, the words her doctor said had her sitting in utter disbelief. He told her she would need to go on kidney dialysis and be placed on the waiting list for an organ transplant.

Because Crystal had always strived to take good care of herself, this really upset her. It was a complication that was out of her hands, no matter how much she did to avoid it. Even more upsetting was wondering how she was going to tell the news to her husband and family!

Denial, Then Relief

Crystal was registered at the University of California–San Francisco (UCSF). Her husband joined her there for her first visit. He wanted to help support her during this difficult first step. Crystal was still having a hard time believing the news and was completely overwhelmed. After meeting the transplant team of surgeons, nurses, staff and faculty, she really allowed herself to let out a sigh of relief. She knew she was in good hands.

She received some excellent news about her condition while there. Crystal learned that she could become a candidate for a new kidney and pancreas, and if successful, she would no longer be diabetic. How incredible that seemed! She had to go through a ton of tests to see if she could handle this type of surgery, and everything tested well. Her years of taking superior care of herself had finally paid off. She was placed on the national waiting list with UNOS.

The Waiting Game

Like many other recipients expressed, waiting on the list was the hardest part, Crystal said. It was such a mix of emotions, just trying to get by day-by-day proved to be difficult sometimes. In a way, she really wanted to hold off on the dreaded surgery, but in another way, she realized her health was deteriorating. She started peritoneal dialysis treatments at home. She was fortunate to be able to do that instead of having to go to a hemodialysis center several days a week for up to 4–5 hours each visit! Doing her dialysis treatments at home gave her quite a bit more freedom, having each treatment last only 40 minutes, done approximately 4–5 times per day. She was able to continue to work and lead a relatively normal lifestyle.

Focus on Inner Strength

Crystal says she always maintained a positive attitude and outlook on life and that nothing could bring her down. She focused on her inner strength to get the transplant and kept reminding herself of the new life that was ahead of her.
✳It had been 1 year and 5 months since she was originally placed on the recipient waiting list. She was not about to give up hope now!✳On November 7, 2000, Crystal was walking in the door to her home, carrying groceries when the phone rang. It was UCSF hospital telling her to get there as soon as possible. She felt such a range of emotions, from joy and relief for herself, to fear and pain in her heart, knowing that another human being had recently lost his or her life. Also, knowing the donor left behind a family, friends, and loved ones was difficult to realize. It was running through her mind constantly. She prayed for the family and silently thanked them for being so gracious in giving the "gift of life."

Good News Posttransplant: Crystal Capser, a 37-year-old Hispanic woman, had a kidney-pancreas transplant after being on the UNOS list for 15 months. Her lab results were so consistently phenomenal at her 1-year posttransplant checkup that she was given a 12–15 year prognosis for life expectancy of the organs and possibly a lot longer! Crystal has been busy as the president of Diabetic Camps for Kids at the Sequoia National Park for 3 years in a row.

Instant Success

Amazingly, the transplant was a complete success and Crystal is doing quite well. The kidney and pancreas began working instantly, without complication. Crystal was, however, extremely sore after her transplant. But she said her energy helped her overcome any of the pain she experienced. She is still amazed at how good she felt so quickly.

I Want to Meet My Donor Family

Crystal was upset about a state mandate by the California Transplant Donor Network regarding meeting donor/recipient families. When she wrote to her donor family, she found that the letters were held up for several months. The donor's family was not told Crystal's information right away because of confidentiality rules. Both parties have to want to seek each other out if they are to ever meet. Otherwise, their information is to be kept to first names only. The families did, eventually, contact each other and meet, and she found out her donor's name was Juan Pedro Namowicz (featured in a sidebar in Chapter 10).

Crystal was afraid the delay of her letter would make her donor's family think she wasn't grateful for the gift. When she was finally able to meet with the family, the Namowiczes, they developed an incredible relationship. Although they ached for the man they lost, they found a friend in Crystal. It helps to have someone in the world that is a reminder of the person they so loved so much.

Another Prayer Answered

One year after her transplant, Crystal met her donor family, which was an answer to her prayers. It was a moment of nervousness and so many other emotions. Her donor's name was Juan, and his entire family came to Crystal's house to visit. They exchanged big bear hugs, tears, and laughter and it was a wonderful visit.

Crystal said, "I could only imagine how the visit must have been for them. I admired their courage. They shared many stories of their loved one, Juan. He left behind a beautiful wife and two young children, three brothers, one sister, his mother, and many other relatives and loved ones. They told of how he made everyone laugh, enjoyed the outdoors, fishing, camping, boating and spending time with his dog." Crystal knew he was an amazing young man who meant so much to everyone whose lives he touched.

It has been 3–and–a half years since her transplant and she considers every day a gift. She thanks Juan for giving her a second chance in life and feels he will live on through her. She will keep him in her heart always. She feels blessed to have his family in her life. They are closer than she ever imagined, and are now her extended family, which she cherishes.

Update: What Is Crystal Capser Doing Now?

Crystal is a volunteer for the California Transplant Donor Network; a public speaker to educate communities (schools, groups, rotary clubs, churches, medical groups, etc.) about the importance of organ donation and sharing how her life has changed since having a transplant; she's a mentor for recently diagnosed diabetics and other patients on the transplant waiting list; and an advocate on the importance for organ and tissue donors.

PERSONAL STORY: ALAN RASKIN—KIDNEY/ PANCREAS RECIPIENT (TYPE I DIABETES— JUVENILE DIABETES)

When Alan was a sophomore in college, he started to have the following symptoms: blurred vision, couldn't concentrate, was always feeling thirsty, and even through he frequently drank water, he'd still have a cottonmouth sensation. He lost approximately 25 pounds without trying and although he often felt dehydrated, he had to urinate frequently.

Alan also had a hard time concentrating. It wasn't until he had problems during intramural basketball season that he suspected something might be wrong. He couldn't even run from one end of the basketball court to the other without having to stop for a drink of water. He decided to stop by the student health center. After suggesting he thought he had mononucleosis, a nurse took a blood sample. By the time he got home for lunch, there was a message asking him to get back to the health center as soon as possible. The message said there was a problem with the test and the center wanted Alan to take it again.

Alan ate lunch, then went back to the health center immediately after. As he waited his turn and saw tons of students come and go, he began to feel uneasy. He was finally told that the doctor wanted to see him and to please just keep waiting. He ended up waiting there for more than 5 hours just pacing between the water fountain and the bathroom. By the time he was finally able to see the doctor he was a complete bundle of nerves and felt nearly out of his mind!

The Diagnosis

As it turned out, the news was worse than he could have imagined. Alan was diagnosed with Type I diabetes. This news was a total shock. He was not prepared for the details that would come next. The doctor told Alan he would have to give himself insulin injections every day—forever—and an ambulance would be there shortly to take him to the hospital.

The doctor said how fortunate it was that Alan had come in on a Monday because it was the only day that he was at the clinic. He was a specialist in endocrinology. The doctor then told Alan that he would be put on a very restricted diet to get his blood sugars under control. He would also have to test his urine several times a day to make sure his sugar levels were consistent.

As if that wasn't enough of a shock, Alan was delivered the most devastating news that not only would he become more susceptible to circulatory and vision problems along with possible heart disease and stroke, but that his life expectancy would be much, much shorter. How is a 19-year-old, all alone with no friends or family with him at that moment, supposed to react or even comprehend such news? As it turns out, he was just so completely overwhelmed that he simply burst into tears.

Considering only hours earlier he had no knowledge of the disease diabetes or what it entailed and now he had a crash course in all the horrors of it, Alan made a life-changing decision. He decided from that point on he would not allow himself to waste his strength or energy asking "why me?" or cry over being diabetic.

Alan considered it a lucky thing that he finally went to a doctor when he did. If he had waited much longer, he may have slipped into a coma and could have died. He did not allow himself to dwell on those horrific thoughts. He just tucked those feelings away. Although he was always aware of those feelings gnawing away at him, he never confessed them to anyone.

A Confusing Description of What Was Happening Inside Him

Alan received news of his disease in 1966. Much more is known about diabetes today. At the time, Alan was given a vague explanation that either his pancreas was not producing insulin anymore, or that if his body was still making insulin it was not being processed the right way.

At the time, it was also believed that Type 1 diabetes was simply inherited. That hardly explained how Alan had gotten it, since he was the first one on either side of his family to have the disease. The real reason that he lost all that weight and was always thirsty was that his body couldn't correctly burn the food he ate. Therefore, it burned fat cells to make up for it.

Alan spent 5 days in the hospital and doctors were able to get his blood sugars where they should be and started him on a very strict diet. He began to feel hopeful again and started to plan his future. He went on to graduate school after college and became a successful businessman in banking. After that, he sold commercial real estate until he landed his dream job as a commodities trader in the pits of the Chicago Board of Trade. It was his lifelong dream to get that job. It also paid him well so he could do whatever he wanted to do in life.

Quick Transition to Adulthood

After a rough transition into adulthood, Alan landed firmly on his feet and was a very happy man. Many years later, in November 1993, Alan received a call from his doctor asking him to come back to redo a blood test. The doctor thought the lab may have made an error and wanted the test redone, just to be safe. That made Alan extremely uneasy because it was just like the call he got in college. He realized that he had suffered from more Type 1 diabetes side effects over the past few years. One specific symptom was losing core vision in his left eye due to damaged nerve and blood vessels.

Unfortunately, the news was worse than the first time, when Alan was diagnosed with diabetes. This time, his results showed he was slipping into kidney failure and would have to be on dialysis. The news was an unbelievable blow to him and was beyond what he could have imagined.

It took years for his kidneys to finally be destroyed, but once his disease had advanced enough, his choices were to either find

a path to the future or do nothing and die. He chose to start
kidney dialysis and to sign up for a transplant. He chose life.

Through the love of family and his then-girlfriend Peggy, he
was able to build a strong support system that allowed him to
be placed on the national organ waiting list.

Alan went through all the stress tests required to see if he
would survive the actual transplant. Because the
kidney/pancreas surgery is usually around a 10-hour operation,
doctors needed to identify possible risks. They found a
blockage of the blood flow to his heart, so they cleared it the
next day with an angioplasty procedure. It wasn't a serious
enough blockage that needed to be fixed if he wasn't going in
for surgery. But doctors corrected it to maximize his chances for
a successful transplant.

Now Alan was healthy and his final details were taken care
of by his transplant coordinator (things like preadmission into
the hospital, arrangement for transportation of donated organs,
change of medications from those that he needed while on
dialysis, to the immunosuppressant drugs he'd need to sustain
his transplant, etc.)

The Transplant

After Alan received his pager, he had two false alarms to go
to surgery (see Chapter 8, "False Alarms Through Transplant
and Beyond"). It was the third call that was the real deal, when
he actually had his surgery. His surgery took place on
Halloween in 1994. It lasted approximately 10 hours, as
doctors predicted, without complication.

Two–and–a half years after his transplant, Alan had an
infection on his right foot. Due to lack of healing, an effect of
diabetes caused by poor circulation and blood vessel and nerve
damage, he needed to have part of his leg amputated, below the
knee. He can walk fine on his prosthetic, so Alan says this
hasn't been an insurmountable problem.

Although it's never an easy road, most posttransplant
problems have not been too much for him to bear. Alan says he
feels better than he has in at least 10 years. Because two people

were kind enough to donate their organs, a kidney and a pancreas, to give him a new life, Alan says, "[he] treats each day as a gift and tries to repay the donors' families by living a full and meaningful life. It is as simple and complex as that."

Update: What Is Alan Raskin Doing Now?

Today, Alan travels to various high schools to tell his story and help spread awareness about the dire need of organ donors. In the 2002–2003 school year alone (when he began speaking at schools), Alan spoke to more than 3,000 high school students! He helps to clear up misconceptions about organ donation. Alan also enjoys writing children's books.

While going through the whole transplant process and recovery, he had two teddy bears that really helped him through his surgery. Their names are Ted and June, and he always takes them with him when he travels.

To read a letter by Alan, discussing his version of his experience in his own words, go to www.giftofhope.org. You can see other recipients' stories there as well.

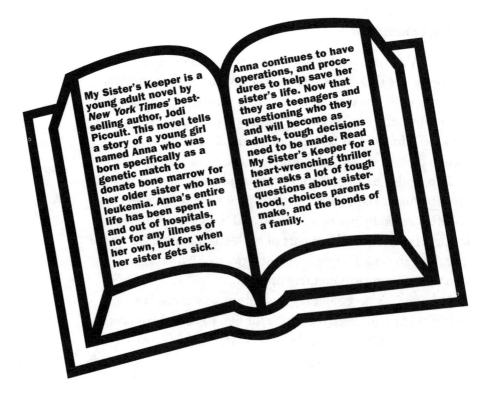

My Sister's Keeper is a young adult novel by New York Times' best-selling author, Jodi Picoult. This novel tells a story of a young girl named Anna who was born specifically as a genetic match to donate bone marrow for her older sister who has leukemia. Anna's entire life has been spent in and out of hospitals, not for any illness of her own, but for when her sister gets sick.

Anna continues to have operations, and proce-dures to help save her sister's life. Now that they are teenagers and questioning who they are and will become as adults, tough decisions need to be made. Read My Sister's Keeper for a heart-wrenching thriller that asks a lot of tough questions about sister-hood, choices parents make, and the bonds of a family.

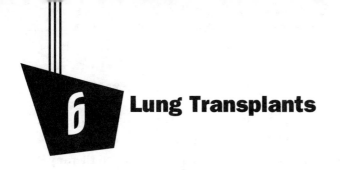

6 Lung Transplants

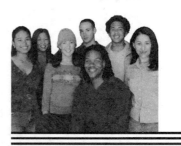

THE TECHNICAL STUFF: Q AND A

Question:
What is a lung transplant?

Answer:
A lung transplant is an operation in which surgeons remove one or both diseased lungs from a person and replace them with a healthy lung(s) from a donor. When speaking of lung transplantation, it could mean a single or double-lung or even a heart-lung transplant.

Question:
Why is a lung transplant needed?

Answer:
The purpose of a lung transplant is to take out a lung or lungs that don't work or are cancerous and replace them with healthy ones from a donor.

Question:
So why can't everyone with a "bad" lung(s) be put on the transplant list?

Answer:
Lungs (and heart) have the shortest life span outside the body of all transplanted organs. They are rare commodities that must be treasured and given out with careful consideration. Far more

people need new, healthy lungs than there are lungs available. To qualify for a lung transplant a person needs to be in end-stage fibrotic lung disease, be dependent on oxygen therapy, and be likely to die of their disease in 12–18 months without a transplant.[1]

?

Question:
Who would be a good candidate for the recipient waiting list?

Answer:
To qualify for a lung transplant, a patient must suffer from severe lung disease that affects their ability to perform regular daily activities or tasks. As mentioned, patients with a life expectancy of 12–18 months or less without a transplant are the ideal candidates for the surgery because they are the most critically ill. Other suitable candidates for lung transplantation are those with: Alpha-1 disease, emphysema, end-stage silicosis, pulmonary vascular disease, chronic pulmonary infection, and cystic fibrosis.[2] However, other considerations are looked at.

Lung Transplant History
1981—first successful heart-lung transplant
1983—first successful single-lung transplant
1987—first successful double-lung transplant.[3]

Patients with emphysema or chronic obstructive pulmonary disease (COPD) who are under 60 years old, have a 2-year or less life expectancy without transplantation, experience progressive deterioration (their health keeps getting worse and worse), and have the emotional stability to deal with the trauma of surgery and aftercare, could be potential recipients.

Young patients with a progressive lung disease, such as end-stage silicosis (see Glossary), are candidates for lung or heart-lung transplants. Patients with Stage 3 or Stage 4 sarcoidosis with cor pulmonale (see Glossary) should be considered for transplantation as soon as possible.

?

Question:

Assuming I am (or my parent is) well enough to be put on the transplant waiting list, what are the risks of surgery and what are typical outcomes of these transplants?

Answer:

Any surgery poses risks, no matter if it is as simple as having your tonsils taken out or as complex as an organ transplant. For transplant patients, the most common and most dangerous complications are organ rejection and infection. The immunosuppressant drugs used to lower rejection pose a risk by allowing a higher rate of infection.

With lung transplants, because the systems involved are so complex and the lungs are fairly fragile organs, the surgery is extracomplicated. Acute rejection usually happens within the first 4 months after surgery, but may even occur years later. An early complication of surgery on the lungs can be poor healing of the bronchial and tracheal openings created during the surgery. A late complication and risk is chronic rejection, which can result in inflammation of the bronchial tubes.

?

Question:

Okay, I'm on "the list" (or my parent is on it) . . . now what?

Overall, lung transplant recipients have demonstrated on average 1- and 2-year survival rates of more than 70%.[4]

Answer:

Once a patient has been selected to be on the list of possible organ recipients, the wait for a matching donor begins. The average wait time for a lung transplant is approximately 1 to 2 years. Obviously, that is just an average. Some recipients wait longer or shorter periods of time, but that seems to be a pretty accurate estimate of how long you or your parent might expect to wait on the recipient list.

Another hard part about waiting, along with not knowing how long it will take, is that the recipient must constantly be available and ready to go to the hospital immediately when a donor match is found. Waiting recipients will be prepared by discussing the exact procedure, risks, expected prognosis, and length of surgery and recovery time with their doctors. They need to continue with all their regular medications and therapies for their disease(s) unless their doctors decide to make alterations.

Although it will be difficult, keeping up your daily routine without huge changes is often best. Not only is your parents' world turned upside-down, but yours is too. Your teen years and beginning adulthood years can be completely stressful without any crazy drama. The medical situation you face as a family going through an organ transplant is a huge deal! See Chapter 7 that focuses on just the "waiting" aspect of the whole transplant scenario.

?

Question:
There's a lung available, so who gets it?

Answer:
When a donor lung(s) does become available, as much information as possible about it is entered into the UNOS computer. Different details are compared between the donor lung and patients on the waiting list. Patients are ranked according to blood type, body size and frame, size of the lungs, and how urgently the person needs new ones to live. Because the lungs (and heart) are the organs with the shortest amount of time to survive once taken out of the donor's body, it is literally a race against the clock.

The blood type is the first and most important component that must match or be compatible. Tissue matching is especially important in lung transplants. The tissues must match as perfectly as possible. After meeting the physical criteria, the waiting patient's health is then considered. Someone might be the sickest person on the list, but if he or she is too sick to survive the surgery, that patient will be passed up. A potential recipient must be stable enough to withstand the intricate surgery, but deteriorated enough to truly need it as a last option.

First, the list of local patients who live within driving distance of the transplant center is checked for a good match. If none are found, the search goes out farther to a regional list.

And if there still isn't a good enough match, the search is opened up to the national list to find the best-matching recipient. The patient's team of lung and transplant specialists makes the final decision to say whether the donor lung is really suitable for the patient. The patient has to be reachable, not have a cold, infection, or other illness, and be ready to get to the hospital immediately.

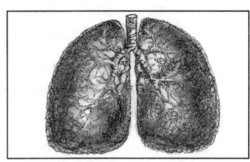

THE ACTUAL SURGERY

While patients are under general anesthesia, single-lung transplants are performed by making an incision in the chest wall, also called a *standard thoracotomy*. Cardiopulmonary bypass is not always necessary for a single-lung transplant.

Lungs remain usable approximately 4 to 6 hours after being removed from the donor. If it is a longer time than that before being placed in a recipient, the lungs could drown from oxygen depletion, causing them to not function properly, or at all.[5]

Because double-lung transplantation involves implanting the lungs as two separate pieces, the bypass is usually required. The patient's diseased lung(s) is taken out and the healthy donor lung(s) are stitched into place. Then drainage tubes are inserted into the chest area to help drain fluid, blood, and air out of the chest. These tubes may stay in place for several days. A double-lung transplant may require a long hospital stay and it could take up to 6 months to recover.

Cardiopulmonary bypass is always needed for a combination heart-lung transplant. A step-by-step process is described in Chapter 3, so please be sure to refer to it there. To do a heart-lung transplant, a cut is made through the middle of the patient's sternum (or breast bone). The heart, lung, and supporting structures are all transplanted into the recipient simultaneously.

This chapter will tell personal stories from two double-lung recipients. The first, Jim Leman, believes his surgery lasted approximately 11 hours. The second recipient, Celeste Morris, said she thought her surgery took approximately 5.5 to 6 hours.

POSTSURGERY: Q AND A

? Question:

What happens right after surgery?

Answer:

Careful monitoring will take place in a recovery room right after surgery and then later in the patient's hospital room. Because the body will consider the new lungs invaders and try to fight them, all transplant patients must take immunosuppression, or antirejection, drugs for the rest of their lives. This will keep the lungs working as if they were original parts of the recipient's body.

? Question:

Are you sure I am (or my parent is) well enough to leave the hospital? I don't know how to take care of medical stuff!

Answer:

Don't worry, whoever received the transplant will most likely have to return to the doctor at least twice a week for follow-up

The outcome of lung transplantation can be measured in survival rates and also improved quality of life for recipients. One study by Gale Group showed that at the 2-year follow-up period, 86% of recipients studied reported no limitation to their activity. That is a huge statement because most had been on full-time oxygen and couldn't perform daily tasks such as dressing themselves, brushing hair and teeth, and so forth.[6]

visits for the first 6 to 8 weeks. The doctors monitor the progress and constantly check on the new organ's function with series of tests.

Your main concern will be to help keep all of your appointments straight, or if your parent had the transplant, you could even drive him or her to appointments, if possible, or perhaps help with the medications. In Chapter 1, I suggest ways to help out by making a binder ahead of time to organize medications taken, reactions, changes, doctor appointments, and so forth.

Question:

How will my family pay for it all?

Answer:

It's important to do research on any and all financial aid available for organ transplants. If your family has medical insurance, it might cover anywhere from 100% of the surgery, to a certain percentage, to none at all. Your parent will most likely be the one looking into those details. (See Chapter 2 for a list of questions to ask regarding finances.)

Because you may be more skilled than your parent on the Internet, or hopefully as knowledgeable because you were raised on it, surf the Internet to find what's out there. In the back of this book is a list of resources to help you begin your search. The United Network for Organ Sharing (www.UNOS.org) has to be one of the best sites when it comes to any organ transplant questions. It has such a wealth of information that I still check in with it monthly to see the current press releases and what's going on in the transplant community, more than 8 years after my father's transplant.

PERSONAL STORY: JIM LEMAN—DOUBLE-LUNG RECIPIENT (CYSTIC FIBROSIS)

Jim Leman is a man who was born with cystic fibrosis (CF), a disease that affects the lungs. In the past, those with CF rarely lived to be older than their 20s. Nowadays, thanks in part to lung transplants, many people suffering with CF are getting a second chance at life. This is the story of one such person.

In 1989, while in the hospital for routine treatment of CF, Jim Leman's doctor said that a lung transplant would become an option for him down the road, in a few years. At the time, Jim didn't believe him and even got angry with his doctor. He felt the suggestion was ridiculous because lung transplants were almost unheard of. Besides, he had a certain comfort in understanding what his body could and could not do. He knew his own strengths and weaknesses. He felt that cystic fibrosis was such a huge part of his life, that it really almost defined him. The thought of risky, experimental surgery frightened him on various levels. Not only was it physically dangerous but also he didn't know what to expect from the outcome.

I Won't Know Who I Am Anymore

What would a lung transplant mean for him? How would his life change, for the better or worse? It was simply too much to absorb. Although he was given the opportunity to ask any questions he wanted, he simply thought the doctors were crazy, so he didn't ask anything.

He was genuinely surprised to hear doctors were already thinking about a transplant. Although his health was bad (breathing wise) Jim generally felt okay most of the time. His doctors even said that he wasn't ready for a transplant yet and to delay it as long as possible. His doctor suggested waiting so that lung transplant technology could improve as much as possible.

In 1995, after another serious setback with cystic fibrosis, Jim knew he was ready to consider transplantation and try to get on the UNOS waiting list. He did get on the list and when he knew his time was close, he asked a lot of questions. Not only did he do a ton of research on the Internet, but he also talked to two or three people who had received lung transplants and another one or two who had heart transplants.

WHAT IS CYSTIC FIBROSIS?

People who have cystic fibrosis (CF) have thick, sticky mucus in their lungs, instead of normal, thin mucus. This mucus blocks the airways and makes breathing difficult. The mucus becomes a breeding ground for bacteria and other infections. One of the most prominent symptoms of CF is the chronic cough, which comes with constant attempts to clear this thick mucus. Continued infections cause damage to the lungs. After too many years of chronic infections, the lungs become too damaged and scarred to do their work.

Some medicines help clear the mucus, but these medicines only work for several hours at a time. Usually a person with CF will have two treatments a day, one in the morning and one in the evening. A person with CF may eventually need supplemental oxygen, at first just at night, then all the time.

Despite continuous use of mucus thinning and clearing medications, as well as antibiotics and physical chest therapy, the mucus will continue to build up and the lungs will slowly become less and less able to function. The person will often become sick and need a week or two in the hospital for more concentrated doses of medicine, IV antibiotics, and more rigorous chest physical therapy. Eventually, despite all efforts, the damaged lungs become unrecognizable and unable to perform. Having lost elasticity, enduring a lifetime of infections and scars, the patient, unable to breathe, will either choose to undergo a double-lung transplant or succumb to the effects of cystic fibrosis.[7] —*Melanie Apel, author, Cystic Fibrosis: The Ultimate Teen Guide*

Okay, It's Worth a Try

Once Jim was being evaluated for the transplant, there was great information and support services for him and his family to cover all aspects of what would be happening each step of the way. Although it was exceptionally frightening for Jim, he said it was probably even scarier for his parents and fiancée, Lisa.

Jim's parents had retired to Arizona 2 years earlier, but about 4 or 5 months before his transplant, they bought a condo approximately 100 yards away from Jim's. They were helpful and supportive. It was a great support system for Jim, and he and Lisa ended up getting married 14 days before his transplant surgery.

When he told Lisa and his parents about considering a transplant, Jim said, "They were stunned, numb, and frightened. It was a little overwhelming and a little hard for us all to comprehend in our hearts."

The answers will differ per family, but here are some questions most families will wonder about:

What is involved in surgery?

How long will it last?

Will there be dietary issues afterward?

What is the percentage of rejection cases?

What about sensitivity to germs because of reduced immune system?

Young adults, especially, have concerns about sexual side effects such as:

Will we still be able to have a family?

Will our intimacy become an issue?

How about the cost of surgery and all the medications I'll be on for the rest of my life?

Will insurance pay for any or all of this?

What about recovery time?

Will I be able to go back to work, and if so, how long after my transplant surgery?

You'll have to discuss these questions with your own practitioner to find the right answers for you.

Team Assigned to Answer All Your Questions

Really tough questions have to be asked including how are the donor organs secured, how is the recipient selected, how do we know the organs are healthy or safe without any tainted blood? Doctors, nurses, social workers, caseworkers, and a team of experts are all assigned to your case to answer any and all of your questions.

Jim was very optimistic and hopeful and tried to minimize any downside. He felt like he had to be a cheerleader around his loved ones. He wanted them to stay as positive as he was.

As mentioned earlier, one of the most difficult parts in deciding to be put on the UNOS waiting list, other than obvious health risks and money strains, was that Jim Leman knew what to expect living his life with cystic fibrosis. He felt it defined him, in part, and learning new limitations or lack of limitations was a very scary prospect to him.

Changing a disease he was used to for a compromised immune system and a life filled with antirejection medications was a prospect he really anguished over, and did not take lightly. In addition to those worries, he feared a transplant might not work.

Although the average waiting time for a lung(s) transplant is 1 to 2 years, Jim only had to wait 8 months. Shortly after receiving his pager, so he could be reached 24 hours a day, he had his surgery. This was, in part, because he got so sick he went to the top of the list (but he wasn't so sick that they took him out of the running). It is a fine line when someone gets gravely ill. In the 8 months he was waiting on the transplant list, he had two interesting "false alarms," which you can read about in Chapter 8.

Jim's surgery took place May 17, 1996, when he was 44 years old. On the way to the hospital, he was rather calm, but very focused. After two false alarms, he and his family had a sharp sense of letdown, exhaustion, and sadness. He had already rewritten his will, and because he worked up until the day of his transplant, he gave his wife Lisa a list of clients to call when he went in for surgery. So his life was pretty much "in order" should he not come out of the surgery.

24/7 Oxygen

By the time he was called for the real deal, he was losing his ability to breathe. Jim was on oxygen 24 hours a day and was constantly fatigued. His operation lasted approximately 11 hours and there were some unforeseen problems. For example, his diseased lungs had lesions that had adhered to his chest. The doctors were able to remove them after much work, but that problem started a series of other unexpected problems. A lung was bleeding, so they had to reopen Jim after the surgery was over, and then a lung collapsed. In the end, the doctors got all of the problems under control and closed Jim up once again. Both of his parents and wife Lisa were in the waiting room while the surgery took place. The first thing Jim remembers after waking up from surgery was his wife's face beside his bed and his dad at the foot of the bed saying, "Hey Jim."

In the first few weeks following surgery, his family treated him almost too delicately according to Jim. They even cooked for him and Lisa, but Jim was way too nauseous (from all the medications) to eat. The nausea continued for quite a long time. (I know that my father still has bouts with nausea and often says things don't smell right or they taste funny. We think it must be from all the medications because he didn't experience this before his surgery.)

The hardest part after the surgery was the recuperation, the effects of the immunosuppressant drugs, and a few rejection setbacks. He had a hard time concentrating because there was a "buzzing" inside his head from the antirejection drugs. Plus, he could not lie flat for more than a month after surgery or else his breathing would stop! Can you imagine having to sleep sitting up all the time?

Jim was self-employed and worried about being off work too long. He went home on IVs because of some complications and had to learn to hook them up himself. Luckily, his wife was able to help out. Doctors, and Jim, wanted him to get back to work as soon as possible. Happily, he was back at work in 30 days.

In the beginning, right after a transplant, it is so difficult for patients to get down the routine of all their medications. Aside from the fact they are achy and tired and recovering from major surgery, the drugs themselves are strong and make concentration quite difficult. I have heard many wonderful stories of how excellent the support staff is in helping patients with their medications. If patients are to recover successfully, they need to

21-YEAR-OLD CF PATIENT MADE AUDIO DIARY FOR NPR STATIONS

First of all, do you know what an NPR station is? When I was in high school, I had no idea, nor did I care what it was. *NPR* stands for *National Public Radio.* (You may have seen a parody of it on *Saturday Night Live.*) It is worth checking out, no matter what your age.

A young woman named Laura Rothenberg suffered from CF. In a *New York Times* article Monday, August 5, 2002, Laura talked about what it was like when she was 12 and 13 years old. She would meet a lot of "CF kids" in the hospital. They really bonded, because they knew what each other was going through. It wasn't something they had to describe or even defend to each other. Most of the kids she knew then have passed away.

Laura was on a cable TV show where teenagers talked about death and a New York radio documentary producer named Joe Richman saw it. He was very moved by her story and mesmerized by her ability to really draw in an audience. He asked her if she'd be interested in making an "audio diary" for NPR.

Over a 2-year span, and many battles with her disease, and an eventual lung transplant that was followed by horrible complications, she gave Mr. Richman a whole series of tapes. He ended up with approximately 15 hours worth of tape that were edited down to a 22-minute program that aired on NPR in 2002.

Laura started raising money and awareness for CF when she was 13. She wanted to educate people about CF and get the word out about organ donation. CF patients can survive past their teens and early 20s now, thanks to lung transplants. In the past, it was rare to live longer than that. In March 2003, Laura lost her battle against CF and died at age 22.

Laura had the idea to make people automatic donors unless they chose not to donate, which is the opposite of how the system is set up now. (You have to request *to* be a donor.) She had an interesting concept that should be taken seriously and explored further.

get that medication routine down pat and have it eventually be second nature to them.

Jim's medical team was great and made him a chart showing what time to take certain pills and how many. This visualization helped him. In fact, his nurse glued each pill next to its name and dosage on the chart. This is a very helpful idea you might want to consider making for yourself (or your parent), with the help of the nursing staff, of course!

Update: What Is Jim Leman Doing Now?

Today, Jim is feeling great and is extremely happy with the outcome of his lung transplant surgery. His insurance covered

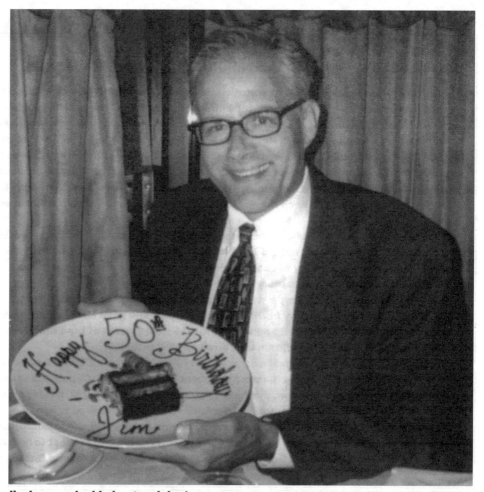

Jim Leman, double-lung recipient

nearly 100% of the bills. His daily life is not affected, and other than the fact he must take medication every day, he really doesn't think about it much, medically.

Jim, like most recipients I've spoken with, says the waiting is the scariest part. You don't know if you'll get a transplant in time. The whole uncertainty of a never-ending wait time is just so difficult. Do your best to use your loved ones for support as much as possible because it will be scary for you, as well. In fact, recipients seem to make peace with either outcome much more so than anxious family members, in my experience.

Jim's final thought for you and your family is, "The [transplant] process can be very successful, but recovery is trying for everyone. Each day has to be taken for its face value. Expect a positive outcome."

PERSONAL STORY: CELESTE MORRIS— DOUBLE-LUNG RECIPIENT (ALPHA-1 ANTITRYPSIN DEFICIENCY)

Celeste Morris was 48 years old when she had a double-lung transplant on September 16, 2002. Her story begins with a routine checkup at Loyola Hospital in Chicago. Celeste has a liver disease commonly called *Alpha-1 disease*. See Chapter 4 for information about the disease.

Some key terms (defined in the Glossary) you might hear regarding a lung transplant are:

Cardiopulmonary bypass
Cor Pulmonale
Immunosuppressive drug
Pulmonary
Pulmonary hypertension
Sarcoidosis
Silicosis

The Alpha-1 Association estimates that approximately one in 3,000 Americans has Alpha-1, but strangely many in the medical community still think of Alpha-1 as rare. Perhaps because 95% of people estimated to have Alpha-1 have not been identified.[9]

Celeste was on the UNOS waiting list for 1 year. How awful it must have been to have such a long wait! However, the average time to wait for a double-lung transplant is between 18 months and 2 years. That is horrifying to learn, especially when waiting for lungs. Take a few seconds to take a deep breath in and out. Do you know how many times you do that each day without even thinking about it? What if each breath were a struggle, or worse yet, had to be assisted by wearing an oxygen cannula?

A Casual Suggestion: Consider a Transplant

While Celeste was at her regular check-up with her pulmonologist (lung doctor), Dr. Patrick Fahey, he suggested she might go talk to the transplant doctors. It was very casual, presented as a suggestion, not something she should absolutely do right away. Therefore, she wasn't really that scared. No one was with her, but she felt comfortable with that suggestion. She was able to ask as many questions from both Dr. Fahey and the transplant team as she wanted. She felt they were very helpful and reassuring.

Because of her Alpha-1 disease, she developed emphysema. It was manageable for years, but as time went on it got more and more unbearable. Not long after she got her pager (to let doctors reach her 24 hours a day) she couldn't even do regular day-to-day things without help, like wash her hair or get dressed. She would become too winded. She had to stop to rest. She received her pager around the first of May 2002, and then didn't have surgery until September 2002.

More Stressful Than You'd Expect—Plan Ahead

Obvious things will stress out a waiting recipient, like "Will I get a transplant in time to save my life?" or "How long will I be on this darned list before I get a healthy organ?" but regular life goes on, not caring what else is happening in your life or anyone else's. Everyday things like a job or stress with your parents, kids, or spouse can get you down. As a teen and young adult, you have exams, a boyfriend or girlfriend, a part-time job, college applications, and tons of other things that might have to be put on hold at a moment's notice, if possible.

Timing is everything, and to show that time waits for no one, 4 days before moving into a new home, Celeste finally got her transplant, after two false alarms (to be discussed in Chapter 8). Not even movers or a mortgage company will wait for a transplant. Celeste had to leave all the work and details to her family. Think of her children, 19 and 23 years old (pictured in Chapter 2); what must have been going on in their lives? They both lived out of state at the time. They probably had to juggle many things to get home ASAP! Plus, Celeste's husband had to ask for help from his friends, in-laws, kids, and anyone else willing to help with his move. Plus, he still had to stay with his wife as much as possible.

It's best to simplify your life as much as possible to avoid getting overly stressed later. You can make a "to do list" in order of importance for projects or obligations you have coming up and mark which ones are flexible and which are mandatory or unchangeable.

If you have a part-time job, you should make your manager aware of your family's situation. Find out if there is room for flexibility in your schedule so you can change or trade hours with another employee when the time comes for your parent's surgery. (If you are waiting for surgery, a part-time job is obviously the last concern on your mind.) You might want to talk to your coworker friends to see if they can be your back up if you need to call them when your parent gets called in for the transplant.

Prejudice

Usually people assume lung transplant recipients have ruined their lungs by smoking heavily. There are so many reasons someone might need a transplant. Yes, they might have been a heavy smoker, however, that's not the only reason for transplantation. Some other examples are diseases like cystic fibrosis and Alpha-1, or a person may have worked in a hazardous field for many, many years (like removing asbestos, coal mining, or working with other hazardous materials).

One thing that so many people are guilty of is prejudice. Not just about a person's race or sex, but even things like how much money a person has or doesn't have, where they live, why they look different, or need a wheelchair, the list goes on and on. Adults do it just as much as kids do, unfortunately.

Celeste Morris said there were times when it was particularly difficult to deal with certain prejudices. For example, when she'd be parked in a handicapped spot at the mall, people would glare at her or even make rude comments. Because she looked like a healthy young woman, people assumed the special parking permit wasn't for her. Once she had to be on oxygen full time, no one thought badly of Celeste using the special parking. But when her illness wasn't obvious just by looking at her, people were often offensive or cruel.

Help From Her Friends

An important part of being a potential organ recipient is that you have a solid support system. That support system will be thoroughly examined while you are still being considered for placement on the UNOS list. A potential recipient's support system is followed up constantly to ensure he or she still has people who will help him or her get through the entire ordeal from waiting for the transplant to posttransplant follow-up care and beyond.

It is equally important that family members have a support system, too. Not that the recipient, your parents, for example, will neglect you, but they might assume that you are uninterested in some of what's going on. Perhaps they will want to shield you from the whole scary situation, so they don't talk about it around you. They might even figure you are self-sufficient enough to take care of yourself, and they won't need to worry about you for a while. That doesn't always happen, but if it does, try not to take it personally.

Hey! A Little Help Over Here, Please!

If you need some attention, speak up and let your parents know. If one of them is the one waiting for a transplant and not you, they might be so wrapped up and consumed by their health and other problems that they are unable to think of anything else. You just have to make your voice heard. Your parents might be afraid to ask you for help, too. If you try to keep talking to each other as much as possible, it'll help keep communication open when it gets more awkward when one of them is really sick and even during the recovery time.

Celeste is married and has two kids. Her sister Ellen came in town and stayed with her to help and to keep her medications straight because Celeste was so drowsy for the first few weeks. She also found great help from her sister Alison and brother-in-law Paul. Paul and Alison's three young children helped to keep Celeste's spirits up by being happy, silly, funny people to be around.

Celeste also says her friends were angels. They went above and beyond the ties of friendship. Her son George and daughter Annie are very close with their parents and knew everything that was going on with their mom's health. Celeste said they were extremely supportive, too. George and Annie even commented on how great their mom's friends were.

In the beginning, it was hard for Celeste to follow the doctor's technical terminology. She didn't know a whole lot about the term *rejection*, other than it was a "bad word." She now knows that it is usually treatable.

To be honest, I didn't know that rejection was usually treatable until writing this book. I always felt "rejection" meant the transplant didn't work, "Stinks to be you. Game over." Please remember: *Rejection is not always the end of the line. It is usually treatable.*

As I have heard from several recipients who have had experienced "false alarms" usually the third time is the real "go." Luckily for me, my father had no false alarms. It isn't like false alarms are routine for everyone, so don't get down or discouraged worrying about that.

Celeste finally got her transplant in September 2002, after being on the UNOS waiting list for just under 1 year. She originally thought she was only going to be a single-lung transplant. But because both donor lungs were healthy, and no other potential recipients were near enough or close enough matches, she ended up having a double-lung transplant. This was extrafortunate for her because it really adds to the quality of life with two healthy, functioning lungs.

Celeste was hearing terms like "1 month out" and "3 months out" by her doctors and was told, "By 1 year out you'll feel back to your old self." She learned that "out" means time that has passed since receiving the transplant. At 8 months "out" now, Celeste says she already feels back to herself. She is amazed at how great she feels.

Education Is Key

When asked if there were any words of advice she'd like to share, Celeste commented, "Yes! Now that I have been through this [transplant experience] I feel strongly that if at all possible, adolescents through young adults should attend an educational/support group through the hospital to share their concerns and also gain understanding of the procedure. They need to see the true picture of what it will be like after the surgery and in the future. . . . I think both of my children (19 and 23 years old) were not given enough information. I think physicians should give this [transplant book] to patients and their families. Children and teens can read it and help get educated about transplantation. It will let them know it will be an emotional time for all."

One of Celeste's biggest concerns was about rehab (getting physical therapy to rehabilitate her body to where she was well enough to leave the hospital and function on her own again). The thought literally exhausted her, but in reality, she learned that it really wasn't so difficult after all, because of her new lungs.

What About Me?

Celeste's son George, who was 19 years old at the time of surgery, and daughter Ann, who was 22 at the time of surgery, shared a lot of thoughts on what it felt like to go through what you, or your parent, are about to go through.

I asked Ann, "What were some of the hardest parts for you during the waiting time, while your mom was on the waiting list?" She said, "It was really hard to keep waiting and see my mother get sicker by the day. She became someone that was not herself. She lost all energy to do daily activities. Another agonizing part was the false alarms we went through."

By Alphas for Alphas
Alpha-1 patients and families have come up with a website "Created by Alphas for Alphas," that you can see on the World Wide Web by going to www.alphanet.org.

All families encounter some family strain during that time. Ann seemed to hint at tension she had with her dad. Because she lived out of state and could not be in Chicago to help her mom, Ann wanted her dad to be more attentive to her mother's needs. She did not seem satisfied with how he handled information. For example, Celeste was admitted into the hospital a few times, and Ann wanted to be there by her side. But her father wouldn't call her until 2 or 3 days into her mother's hospitalization. That usually meant her mom would be released soon after, so Ann wouldn't have time to get home, or wouldn't need to bother at that point.

When reading her questionnaire about the experience, it seemed as though Ann felt very isolated. She said her father was the one person who could have reacted or done something about her feelings regarding the situation. However, he was not at all responsive to her or her feelings.

If your parent acts like that too, kind of withdrawn from you or the entire situation and the other parent, it will feel awful. But try to think of what it must be like from that parent's point of view. Not only would he or she be left to raise you alone, but would also lose his or her partner and best friend.

I Won't Miss You If I'm Mad at You

For some people, it is easier to be mean, pick a fight, or try to be mad at someone who might die than to keep hope alive and stay positive and hopeful. It is a natural human response of "fight or flight."

Luckily, Ann had great friends to help her with the whole ordeal. She even had a longtime family friend who flew home with her from Florida to Chicago to be with her through the hard times.

Other than the basic fears and questions most kids and other family members have, such as "How long is the actual surgery? What are the dangers of surgery?" Ann's biggest fear was her mother dying. She says her mom is the closest person to her. Happily, Celeste is alive and healthy and enjoying her family thanks to the kindness of strangers who donated lungs so life can go on for others.

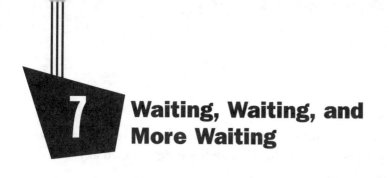

7 Waiting, Waiting, and More Waiting

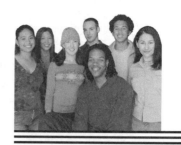

REAL ANSWERS FOR YOUR DEEPEST, DARKEST QUESTIONS

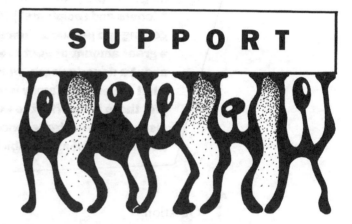

This is quite possibly the most important chapter for young adults to read. Many questions will cross your mind and might even make you feel bad for thinking them. *Don't!* Don't feel bad for any thoughts you have; they are completely normal when faced with life or death situations. Some of these are questions I asked myself, and usually dared not mention to anyone else, not even to my brothers and sisters. The other questions are some that you might be thinking.

The questions below, which vary from overnight trips to wedding plans, show various perspectives of different aged "kids/young adults" who have a loved one about to get a transplant or who are even waiting for one themselves. What is important to remember is that *your life must go on*, no matter what the status of your loved one's transplant schedule. You cannot put your life on indefinite hold.

BEFORE SURGERY: TECHNICAL STUFF[1]

? Question:
Who can be a donor?

Answer:

Anyone, regardless of age, race, or gender can become an organ and tissue donor. Medical suitability is determined after the donor's death.

Why are the terms used so cold and technical? The transplant community uses impersonal language (i.e., "harvest" organs, "donors and recipients") to avoid getting too personal. Since there is a great amount of guilt in knowing about a donor's death, which may be what saved your family member's life, there is an effort to keep the discussions as sterile, anonymous, and as minimal as possible.

? **Question:**

I've heard the term "living donor" and wondered what does that mean, and what other kinds of donors are there?

Answer:

A living donor has given part of an organ (liver, lung, or pancreas) or one kidney from his or her own living body for transplantation, usually to a family member. A living donor's other kidney can do the work of the two kidneys. Because kidneys are matched genetically, a family member donating to another family member tends to be a much more successful match than one from an unrelated donor.[2]

The other kind of donor is cadaveric donor, which means the person has died. That is what you volunteer to do by signing your driver's license. It's like you saying, "I don't mind if someone uses my organs when I'm gone." When at a support group meeting once, I got a really cute button that said, "Don't Take Your Organs to Heaven. Heaven Knows We Need Them

Here." I kept it and still wear it sometimes. It usually gets people's attention and they ask about it. Then I tell them how an organ donor saved my dad's life.

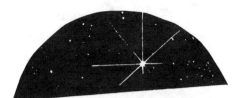

? Question:
What organs and tissues can be donated?

Answer:
The liver, heart, lungs, kidneys, pancreas, corneas, bone, saphenous veins, heart valves, small intestine, and skin are some of what can be donated.

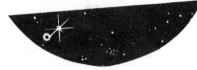

Don't Take Your Organs To Heaven Heaven Knows We Need Them Here.

? Question:
Being a living person, can I help by donating something like blood, bone marrow, or a kidney?

Answer:
If a person is healthy and matches the medical criteria, he or she can be a donor. There is not an age limit, although persons younger than 18 years old need to have a parent's or legal guardian's written permission.

? Question:
Why do I have to tell my family over and over again that I want to be a donor? I signed my driver's license, isn't that enough?

Answer:
No, if you sign your donor card, your family still needs to know about it. If something happens to you, your family will be asked to sign a consent (permission) form for donation to take place. If they don't sign it, the organ procurement organization cannot use your gift.

? Question:
What if I change my mind after I get a donor card and don't really want to do it after all?

Answer:
Just tear up your card and tell your family that you do NOT want to be a donor. Again, your family has to sign a consent form. They get the final say if you become a donor or not.

? **Question:**

Are you sure doctors will still do their best to save my life if I have a signed donor card?

Answer:

Yes, absolutely. The transplant team has no involvement in a patient's care before death and is only notified after death has occurred. The doctor's job is to save their patients, so you are their number one concern!

? **Question:**

If I donate my organs, will I look gross so my family can't have a funeral?

Answer:

No, any organs and tissues donated are removed by a surgical procedure. It is done neatly so that any regular funeral arrangements (like open-casket wake) can be made.

? **Question:**

What organs and tissues are most needed?

Answer:

Corneas and kidneys are needed most in terms of the number of people waiting. But if you're talking about organs needed to save a life, hearts, lungs, and livers are needed the most.

? **Question:**

Are there costs to donate organs and tissues?

Answer:

There is no cost to the donor's family or estate. All costs associated with the donation are covered by the organ procurement organization (OPO). The medical costs of treating the patient, up to the point of donation, are still the responsibility of the family. Organ donation is a gift and it is illegal in the United States to buy or sell organs or tissues.

? **Question:**

How long can it be before the organs have to come out of the donor? Do they "go bad"?

Answer:

Organs must be removed as soon as possible after the person dies so they can still remain useful. Here's an example of how fast an organ should really be placed into a waiting recipient. Then you can see how precious the gift is and why people have to get right to the hospital when they get called for a transplant.

Heart/lung—between 4 to 6 hours

Pancreas—between 12 to 24 hours

Liver—up to 24 hours

Kidneys—48 to 72 hours

Corneas—must be transplanted within 5 to 7 days

Heart valves, skin, bone, saphenous veins—may be preserved from 3 to 10 years.[3]

Question:

Does a person's race matter? Can whites, African Americans, Native American, Asians all donate to each other?

Answer:

Organ size is one of the most crucial things to match up between donor and recipient when a heart, liver, and/or lung(s) are being transplanted. But genetic makeup is especially important when matching kidneys; so the better "match" will be a kidney donated from a person of one race to another person of the same race.

Question:

Who decides who gets organs and when? For example, do celebrities or politicians get "special treatment?"

Answer:

No, there is no way to "cheat the system." A huge variety of factors are taken into consideration, such as blood and tissue typing, how long the patient has been on the waiting list, geographical locations of possible donors and possible recipients, and most important, medical urgency—how sick the potential recipient is. Organ donations are organized by UNOS and it handles the entire organ donor list for the United States.

WHILE I'M WAITING: PERSONAL AND EMOTIONAL STUFF

? Question:

Why do I feel so mad at my mom for being sick? In my head, I know it's not her fault, but my heart is so angry with her!

Answer:

Your parent is sick and may need taking care of, or at the very least, is not able to totally take care of and focus on you like he or she usually does. "But that's a parent's job," you might think, "to be here for *me*."

Families are made to take care of each other. Instead of being angry all the time, try and think how your parent must feel. If your dad is the sick one, he might feel like a failure for not spending all his energy on you and what's going on in your life, or perhaps he gets scared about what will happen to you if he does not make it. He has so many things to worry about, so try to think of it from the angle of being "honored" or "proud" that he now depends on *you* for some help and support. That is something you weren't old enough to provide in the past, and you can feel responsible or at least more grown up, for doing your part for the family.

> **Good Advice From a Teen Who Has Been There**
> "It is so important to set up your own support system. Having a person you can say absolutely anything to without feeling selfish or negative or bitchy or scared is something that will get you through this awful time!" —Lisa, 18 year old

? Question:

Should I still stay overnight at friend's house or just stay close to home all the time?

Answer:

Assuming you parent isn't in some form of crisis (i.e., total liver failure or some other serious problem), where a transplant might be necessary that night, yes, go to a friend's house. A sleepover might give you the fun you need to take your mind off your parent and let you relax and do something besides worry.

? **Question:**

Should I be a summer camp counselor (at a camp far away from home) this year, or just stay close?

Answer:

This decision is very personal. Although it is important to maintain some sort of stability in your life, going away from your family for several weeks might add to your stress. Maybe you've been so worried for so long and the camp is only an hour away and you could get home quickly if anything should happen. If that is the case, it might do you a world of good to take a break and get away by yourself. You could even consider a shorter camp obligation for a week or two instead of for the whole summer.

? **Question:**

Should I still go on my class trip?

Answer:

You need to evaluate your decisions on a day-by-day basis. But if your parent has been doing really well and has no big changes coming up (i.e., new medication or procedures), a 3- or 4-day field trip might be just what you need to regroup and renew the hope and encouragement needed to keep your loved one's spirits up.

> *Reputable Sources or Not?* "Be sure to check out where your Internet information is coming from. A teacher once told me 'dot com' could be given to any self-proclaimed expert. But websites ending in '.org' or '.gov' are websites that are monitored by professionals in a particular field. That doesn't mean all 'dot com' websites stink, some solid information can be found on them, but it just isn't necessarily monitored for its accuracy."
> —Lisa, 18 years old

? **Question:**

Should I apply to college, or take a year or two off to be close to home?

Answer:

Usually, it is not recommended that huge life plans, such as college be put on hold. But, as always, you need to go with your gut feeling for this decision. You might want to alter your plans and hold off going to some school several states away and go to a school closer to home. You could even stay at home and attend a community college for the first year or two and fill your general educations requirements. Such a large decision should be made as a family. It's best to consult your parents before rejecting any acceptance letters from universities.

AFTER SURGERY: I CAN'T ASK THESE QUESTIONS—I SOUND TOO SELFISH

? Question:
Will I ever get over it if something bad happens in surgery?

Answer:
Again, I cannot stress how important some sort of support system is for every member of the family! You are young and need to turn to friends, but also to some adults, whether it is your other parent, a teacher, or even a friend's parent. Hopefully, by now, you are a member of a support group through the hospital with other families going through the same things you are. It will really help you to not feel so alone.

? Question:
Will my mom survive such a loss emotionally, or just be completely sad forever?

Answer:
Although your family members might feel the world has stopped and they won't be able to get out of bed to see another day, life does go on. That's the whole premise of organ transplantation. Hopefully, by others giving the gift of life, your loved one will get the transplant that is so desperately needed!

Adults have usually dealt with death more than kids, so they have some experience with it. It won't lessen the grief, but most people know that with time, things do eventually get better. Talking to a professional counselor and/or support group is so important to a family before, during, and after a transplant. There is another book in the It Happened to Me series, on grief and loss, by Edward Myers that you might find helpful, too. It is titled *When Will I Stop Hurting? Teens, Loss, and Grief: The Ultimate Teen Guide*.

Question:

Who will take care of us financially? (Will my mom be able to take care of me and pay all the bills herself?)

Answer:

Many people have some sort of life insurance. If this is the case, money won't be of immediate concern. However, if life insurance isn't something your loved one had in place before, all of your family members may need to pull together to go over a budget. Together, you can figure out ways for everyone to take part to cut back expenses and pitch in to earn some extra money. It's especially hard for teens making minimum wage, or if you aren't old enough to get a real paying job, you could do something as simple as babysitting or a paper route that can add up quickly to meet *your* wants or small needs. This way, you won't get tempted to ask for money for the latest CDs or to go out with friends. You can pay for your "fun stuff" yourself.

You will probably find that you will stop buying a lot of the stuff you feel you just *have* to have once it comes from the money that took you such a long time to earn.

"Uh . . . Bye!" A recipient named Jim was literally about to walk out on stage to be a keynote speaker at a conference when his pager went off. He simply said, "Excuse me, I have to leave," and he went right to the hospital. He is a perfect example of bad timing, but also of someone who is willing to leave at a moment's notice no matter what.

? Question:

Who will take care of us and keep all our schedules straight? (If mom doesn't get the transplant in time and dad has to work all the time, who will get us after sports practice or take us to work, and so forth? Will we just have to give up all our extracurricular activities?)

Answer:

Your dad is going to need to be close with you now more than ever. He'll want to know the details of your life because he can only get that information from you. Fathers need as much love and support as their kids do, so don't write him off so quickly. Dads can be equally nurturing, if not more so, than some mothers.

? Question:

What if my dad survives the surgery but takes a lot longer to recover than anticipated? (Will he lose his job? Will he ever be able to physically return to work?)

Answer:

The United States has a law called Family and Medical Leave Act that requires a company to hold a job for someone for up to 12 weeks (unpaid) who is physically unable to work for an extended period of time. Although they might have to temporarily or permanently replace the position your parent had, the company is legally required to have some job available upon his or her return. You can read the actual act by going to http://www.dol.gov/elaws/ esa/fmla/sl.asp.

? Question:

My boyfriend and I just got engaged. Should I move up my wedding date and cancel my honeymoon?

Answer:

This was a question I dealt with myself. As some of you are in your late teens or 20s, you might be engaged. Personally, I kept my plans as originally made, although doctors predicted my father had approximately 1 year to live without a transplant, and my wedding was still several months away. My father lived to walk me down the aisle (with his pager on his tuxedo cummerbund!). Looking back at pictures, he really looked on death's door, but at the time, I couldn't see it. I still lived with my parents and saw him every single day, so I didn't notice the gradual changes that were happening each day.

Taking a honeymoon was a tougher decision because I was planning to go to Mexico, but I ended up going. These days, almost anywhere you go is a plane ride away. My brother Jerry, who lives in Australia, hopped on a plane immediately upon hearing of my dad getting a new liver and still made it to the hospital before my dad was coherent enough to have visitors. (Remember, most transplant surgeries are *very* long!)

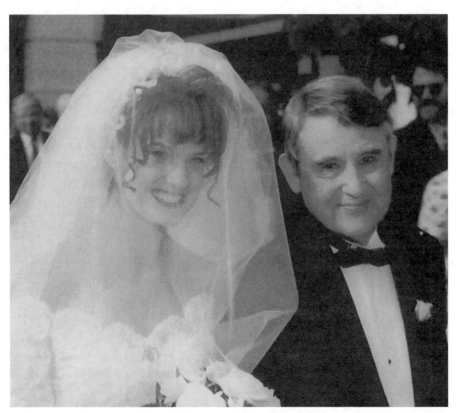

Jim Purcell, liver recipient, walking daughter down the aisle of her wedding wearing his pager (not shown)

? Question:

Will my dad, or even me, if I'm the one getting the transplant, look or feel different with someone else's organs inside him (me)?

Answer:

Of course, he (or you) will feel different! After months of serious recuperation and hard work, he (you) will hopefully feel like a new and healthy person. As far as feeling literally like a new person, people have made different statements on the subject. For example, in the movies people often say things like, "I never liked pickles my entire life, now I want pickles every day." I'm not sure how much of that is true, but there is documentation of some mild similarities. However, things like a criminal or "bad guy" living through a person is completely untrue. Those are things moviemakers do in horror movies to scare you!

? Question:

Because someone had to die for my dad to get a transplant (true for some liver patients and all heart patients), can I write to the family to say thank you?

Answer:

Organ donation is anonymous, which means you are not given the name of the donor or the family. However, you *can* write a letter and have your transplant coordinator send it to the procurement agency that will forward it on to the family of the donor (as shown in the movie *Return to Me*, featuring Minnie Driver and David Duchovny).

I wrote a letter thanking the donor family and let them know how grateful I was that my dad would live long enough to see me have children and my kids would know my dad (their grandpa) thanks to their gift of life.

? Question:

Will we get any information on the donor?

Answer:

We were only told my dad's liver was donated by a man in his 40s who had a heart attack while jogging. We don't know if he was married or had kids. I think that knowledge is too difficult for patients to know. For example, I can never talk to my dad about it, but I remember sensing his uneasiness about the whole subject of the donor. There is a terrible feeling of guilt people have knowing someone needed to die in order for them to live.

There is debate going on about whether donor families and recipient families should meet. Initially, after the surgery, you can write a letter just using your first name and the transplant coordinator will send it to the procurement agency, who will forward it on to the donor family. If the donor family wishes to respond or seek you out, then the coordinator will forward a note from the family to you. Then you may exchange names, write to each other, and perhaps even call or meet.

A recipient named Crystal Capser, featured in Chapter 5, discusses how she and her donor family met and developed a relationship. It was the same with the Green family, highlighted in Chapter 10, but I think that happens with a smaller percentage of people and is not the norm. It is a subject really being "tiptoed" around for now.

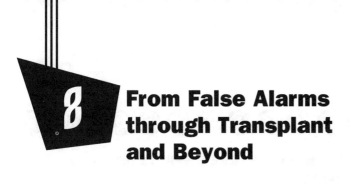

From False Alarms through Transplant and Beyond

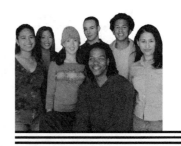

FIRST THING TO REMEMBER: BE HAPPY FOR EVERYONE WHO DOES WELL IN SURGERY

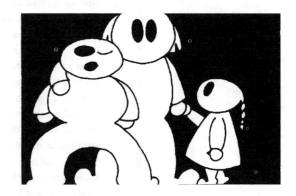

As a recipient or family member, it's good to remember a few things while waiting for a transplant. Remember to support others who are going through this experience. It sounds impossible, but even setbacks like getting passed up by someone lower on the list or someone who was added after you or your parent is not something to hold a grudge about. Some people simply match up more perfectly with a donor than (you or) your parent does. Many things have to match besides just a blood type. Tissues, blood, body type, even ethnic or similar nationalities can help make a more perfect match.

I remember sharing the waiting room with a family during my dad's surgery. Granted, we were there for countless hours (around 13–15 hours, because my dad had a ton of scar tissue from previous surgeries that really slowed things down, and doctors can't estimate such delays). The other family had a mom in for a multiple-organ transplant. We half-jokingly fought over what TV shows to put on and who got the couches and who got the floor. I vividly remember being extremely jealous of that family.

WAYS TO KEEP EVERYONE'S SPIRITS UP WHILE WAITING

- Remember, any organ that gets "passed up" by surgeons is turned away with your (or your family member's, depending on who is waiting for the transplant) best interest in mind. With the shortage of organs, the team of doctors needs to be sure a recipient has the best chance of survival and recovery.
- The long road to recovery will be challenging. There is no room for negative thoughts. Rely on each other to keep spirits up in the family or support-group situation.
- Try to use the waiting time to plan ahead. Suggest making a three-ring binder to organize everything from medications to a journal of thoughts, feelings, photos, progress, and so forth after the transplant. You and your parent could have fun together making the journal bright and colorful. You could mix the scary stuff, like the numerous medications needed, each organized and defined, and the dosage amount documented with milestone charts of how each day your parent (or you) improved and felt better and better.
- Even taking a picture every few days or weeks that shows you or your parent's progression will serve as a great reminder of how far the patient and family have come together throughout this whole ordeal.

Only hours after surgery, their mom was awake, alert, playing cards, and joking around with them. My dad wasn't even out of surgery yet. Once he was finally out of surgery, he was so whacked out from the anesthesia and morphine that he acted crazy, even hours later. He was trying to rip off his hospital gown because he was hot (and my mom was mortified because he was totally naked under his gown). I still laugh about that one! Here the poor guy has had his guts ripped out and replaced and has literally cheated death, and my mom is worried about Dad flashing us or some intensive care nurses who've seen it all before. Crazy!

SOME THINGS YOU'LL ACTUALLY
LAUGH ABOUT . . . SOMEDAY

Some silly things happened that I remember fondly, but were pretty serious at the time. My dad and I joke about certain things between us, but out of respect for the other family members' feelings, we try not to talk about it in front of them.

As my dad was slowly coming out of his fog and haze of pain medication, my brother Jerry, who lives in Australia, arrived to see him. We were all getting pretty positive, thinking dad might just come out of this after all. For a while, I was afraid perhaps he had suffered brain damage or something! Your mind can wander to all sorts of horrible scenarios when faced with scary situations and although brain damage was never mentioned, we all were a bit sleep deprived and crazy ourselves.

An important thing to remember is, no matter whether you and your family went through a transplant last week, or 10 years ago, or are still waiting in limbo to get one, some people just cannot revisit the emotions of it all. It is simply too painful, and they'd rather not discuss it ever.

My mom, dad, and I can all talk about my father's transplant pretty freely, but I rarely discuss details with my four siblings. That is just how it panned out in my family. It is still an emotional subject for the majority of them. I didn't even realize, myself, how many of them are still dealing with it until I wrote this book.

A HORRIBLE SHOCK

The family whose mom was doing so well took a strange and immediate turn for the worse two days after surgery and died unexpectedly. My family was devastated. We felt like friends on a battlefield, bickering and joking together through one of the roughest times in our lives. We were strangers thrown together, becoming friends out of necessity.

To this day, I feel guilty about the jealousy I felt toward that family and its members. I remember it so clearly. I've asked myself hundreds of times, "*Why* couldn't I just be happy for them, why?" It wouldn't have made my dad's recovery time any longer if I was happy for their good fortune. I was selfish with my jealousy and now my parent is alive and theirs isn't.

That is why it is so important to be positive for your family and the other families in the transplant community. If you go to support groups and other people only had to wait a week for a transplant while your parent has been on the list for nearly a year and has failing health, don't begrudge the other's good fortune. It's a waste of your energy and will only make you feel bad later. There are many opportunities for regret in the whole transplant scenario, so don't add possible situations to the list.

What A Team! You would be amazed at just how many people make up an actual "transplant team." It is so much more than the surgeons and nurses! A few members of the team include the transplant coordinator, anesthesiologists, social workers, the surgeons and nurses, rehabilitative therapists, insurance people, and administrative staff.

FALSE ALARMS VERSUS THE REAL DEAL

Crystal Capser: Kidney/Pancreas Recipient

Crystal is one of the recipients discussed in Chapter 5. After receiving her pager, she was paged several times. Confused, she finally discovered that the pagers given to waiting recipients are donated (usually from a place called LifePage, www.nepaging.com/lifepage.htm) and are refurbished, or used, pagers. She had a pager that belonged to someone else a few days earlier.

Although it is frowned upon, the person who had the pager before her used it like a regular pager and gave the number out to friends and family who would frequently call to check in. It is recommended that only the transplant coordinator have the pager number. The news that someone else now had the pager didn't seem to get around very quickly, so Crystal kept getting calls for the previous owner by mistake.

The first time Crystal received a page, her heart nearly stopped. She was so nervous and jittery to answer the call, but it was a false alarm. After a couple of these calls, she was less nervous to return them. In fact, she didn't want to call the numbers after a while, for fear that it was another message for the person who used to have it. That caused her anxiety and frustration. But she had to return every call because she never knew whether the number would be the real one, so she continued to return five "mistake" calls!

Finally, Crystal's turn came to get the "real call" from the transplant coordinator. The ironic part is that he reached her at home by telephone. She didn't even need to be paged. She ended up receiving a combination kidney/pancreas transplant. Although it was extremely difficult and painful, there were no surgical complications. Her surgery was 3 years ago, and today she feels great, like a woman with a new lease on life.

Celeste Morris: Double-Lung Recipient

Celeste Morris also experienced false alarm calls, but ones quite different from Crystal. Celeste received a double-lung transplant after spending almost 12 months on the UNOS list. During that time she had two false alarms. These were calls for her to go to the hospital for her transplant. When she went to the hospital for the very first time, she thought, "This is it." But surgeons disagreed after finding not only one of the donor lungs had trauma to it, but there was extensive damage to both lungs, so neither could be used.

Celeste was called in for surgery a second time, and again the donor lung was in such bad shape, doctors would have only used it if she were actually dying at the time. It may have been used as a last resort to keep her alive until a better one was available, but luckily that was not her situation.

When Celeste got the real call that gave her the new set of healthy lungs she so desperately wanted and needed, her surgery went on without complication and she is alive and well now, almost a year after surgery. She says she feels better than ever, so the emotional strain of the false alarms was worth it in the end. (See photo of Celeste with her husband and two kids in Chapter 2.)

When discussing false alarms, I've heard some recipients say they were a bit relieved not to have to go through surgery right then, that fear was a bit of a consolation. Having a transplant surgery called off is an emotional let down, to put it mildly, but to have to go through that roller coaster more than once can be unbearable!

After two false alarms, Celeste and everyone else in the family were on edge, especially her husband. In addition to the unbelievable stress, their house was being remodeled and the dust was really irritating her lungs. They decided it best if they moved into a hotel until the house was done or she had the transplant, whichever came first.

When families have to fly in for the surgery, another stress of unknown timing is added to the list. (See the sidebar about the way TRIO can help with some of the stress you and your family may be feeling.)

As mentioned in an earlier chapter, if your parents don't get along well during the wait or after the surgery, don't feel like you're the only one to experience this. *You are not alone.* Families have to really work hard to keep it together and survive the whole ordeal. Transplant situations put a tremendous amount of strain on the entire family. That strain can break the family apart if everyone isn't 100% able to keep working on staying together.

Family troubles are part of why having a transplant is not a choice everyone simply jumps at. Some people choose to forgo a transplant altogether, even if it means the only hope of their survival. It brings up the debate of quality of life versus quantity of life again. In Chapter 12, on regrets, you'll see that some people

TRANSPLANT RECIPIENTS INTERNATIONAL ORGANIZATION, INC.

TRIO, which stands for *Transplant Recipients International Organization, Inc.*, is a wonderful organization that helps families in the transplant community. Each year, TRIO accepts applications for its scholarship program. The program gives thousands of dollars in academic grants to members and their families.

In 2001, ten $1,000 scholarships were given to deserving students who are transplant candidates, recipients, their family members, and/or donor family members. Various TRIO chapters donated the money along with separate individuals and interested organizations.[1] If you'd like to apply for their yearly scholarship or make a donation to the fund call TRIO at 1-800-TRIO-386, or e-mail them at info@trioweb.org.

Another great contribution TRIO makes toward transplant families is giving airline miles that have been donated to help transplant recipients get to the centers far from home, or to help other family members fly in for the transplant so they can all be together. The TRIO website has a wealth of great information, www.trioweb.org. Check it out!

who have had a transplant ultimately regret it. (Two examples in that chapter involve a hand transplant recipient and someone with unforeseen complications from cystic fibrosis.) That's why deciding whether or not to have the surgery is a very serious decision that requires a lot of thought and discussion.

By reading this book, you've already taken an important step by educating yourself with technical information and personal stories of what it'll really be like for you and the whole family. That's a really big deal and you should feel proud of yourself for taking charge of your situation and not just acting like a victim of some horrible circumstance.

Jim Leman: Double-Lung Recipient

On January 28, 1996, Jim Leman was seconds away from leading a seminar in Chicago. As he was about to walk on stage to address the crowd, his pager went off. He literally had to walk out, introduce himself, then say, "Excuse me for the last minute notice, but I have to leave," and that was it, he left. This happened 4 months after being added to the UNOS waiting list to get a new, healthy pair of lungs, after suffering from cystic fibrosis since birth.

Unfortunately, when he got to the hospital, he found out that the donated lungs were not healthy and functioning properly, so the surgery was called off. His entire family was devastated.

Three months later, after being on the transplant waiting list for a total of 7 months, Jim got a call at 9:30 P.M. on April 12, 1996. Again, he raced to the hospital, along with his fiancée Lisa and his mom and dad. They got all the way to downtown Chicago, to Loyola University Hospital, only to find out the quality of the donated lungs was not good and the surgeons elected not to operate. The emotional roller coaster was almost too much to bear. Luckily, they managed to pull together and find strength in one another to psych themselves up to be put back on the waiting list.

Some great websites now offer support and guidance for dealing with the emotional trauma of the highs and lows while waiting on "the list" (see sidebar).

www.transweb.org "Trans Web: All About Transplantation and Donation" is a nonprofit educational website based at the University of Michigan whose mission is to serve as a resource for patients, families, students, health care professionals, and the general public, as well as to promote organ and tissue donation. When the site launched in January 1995, Trans Web was the first transplantation and donation website in the world.

Finally, on May 17, 1996, Jim got "the call" and knew that "the third time's the charm!" Sure enough, he was right. After having two false alarm calls, he and his family had a sharp sense of let down, exhaustion, and sadness, but they went off to the hospital feeling full of optimism.

Jim was prepped for surgery, which was 14 days after his wedding to Lisa, and then he was wheeled away for his double-lung transplant. The surgery took approximately 11 hours, and he came through fine with only a couple of complications. Because his sick lungs had lesions on them, they stuck to his chest wall like glue. Doctors were able to get them off and out of Jim's body to put in the new lungs. One of the new ones bled when the surgery was done, so they had to reopen Jim, causing one lung to collapse. Before long, the surgeons had everything under control, pumped up, and in working order. They closed Jim up and he was good as new.

After coming out of the anesthesia, one of the first things Jim remembers is seeing his wife's face beside his bed. His dad was at the foot of the bed and simply said, "Hey Jim." The hardest part was over and it was a big sigh of relief for all of them.

Alan Raskin: Kidney/Pancreas Recipient

Five months after Alan received his pager, it went off one night at 12:30 A.M. He was sleeping and was hooked up to a home-dialysis machine. He knew before even answering the phone that it was his transplant coordinator, Doug. Doug was disappointed when Alan told him that he had developed an infection at the site where his catheter was inserted, and that he was on antibiotics. Doug was frustrated that Alan did not keep him informed. Infection temporarily disqualifies a waiting recipient. Alan would have to wait until his infection was gone and he had been off antibiotics for 2 weeks before being considered for transplantation again. Although a bit upset, Alan was not really devastated because he was moving up the list.

Alan's next call came in September on a Sunday afternoon. He went to the hospital for his preoperative testing. Everything was going well until the resident came to tell him the donor kidney was not functioning right. The surgery was called off at 5:30 P.M. As the resident left, he told Alan that the surgery would have been canceled anyway because the pre-op physical showed he had signs of internal bleeding. Alan was so angry, mostly with his own body. He started to feel that for every step he took forward, he had to take two steps back. What calmed his frustrations and allowed him to hang in there was the love of his family and of his girlfriend, Peggy. That's the perfect example of why the transplant team makes sure there is a strong support system in place, otherwise setbacks like Alan faced might give waiting recipients such a bad attitude that it would compromise the whole situation.

The third time Alan's pager went off, he knew it was the transplant coordinator, Doug. Other than Peggy, whose house Alan had just left, Doug was the only one with his pager number. This third time around was the real deal. As Alan spoke to Doug about what time to arrive at the hospital, he started shaking. His adrenaline was pumping and he wasn't able to stop shaking until he was given a sedative on the way into surgery.

Although there was a mixture of excitement and fear on his part, he was truly concerned about what would happen to his family and Peggy if he didn't survive. He felt he led a great life and was prepared for any outcome. In fact he said he picked out the music for his funeral on the way to the hospital, just in case. He wasn't being negative. Alan just wanted to spare his loved ones any suffering he could if he died. He wanted them to celebrate his life and focus on the good in it.

Happily, the surgery went great, and 10 years later, Alan is still alive and well. Although he's faced challenges, as all candidates and recipients do, Alan says, "None of the challenges have been insurmountable. I live each day to the fullest, mostly out of respect and gratitude to the donors and donors' families."

Jim Purcell: Liver Recipient

Jim Purcell, whose story was highlighted in Chapter 4, almost didn't get to go through with his planned surgery because of a very low-grade fever. Fortunately, it was so low that it posed no risk of infection or illness, so he was able to go through with the operation on the first try. He had no "false alarms" to speak of.

When Jim was called, he was home alone without anyone to drive him. His wife was out, none of his grown kids were at their homes, and I, his only daughter still living at home with my parents, was at a baptism 30 miles west of where he was. Jim had to call some friends to take him from the northern suburbs to the south side of downtown Chicago, where the University of Chicago hospital is located.

My sisters-in-law and I remember vividly how we had all just sat down for my nephew Griffin's baptism when my pager went off. It was my brother's wife on the phone telling me dad was on his way to the hospital and to get there as soon as possible. I ran out of the church alone, crying, not even knowing how to get to the hospital. I'd been there many times before, but always sitting in the back seat reading a book while my mom and dad chatted and/or bickered on the way to the support group meetings, which was a stressful place to visit at times. I never paid attention to the driving directions.

I've always been a nervous passenger in cars, so if I'm not driving, I prefer to read. There I was, driving blindly on the expressway and I decided to call Sue Raucher, one of my best friends since high school, to ask directions. She had moved to Arizona with her family after graduation, but once dated a guy who went to the University of Chicago. I thought she might know the way. What a crazy idea that was—how the heck would *she* remember? (She wouldn't even drive on the expressway herself until she was in her 20s!)

Sue put her dad on the phone and he tried to calm me down and get me there in one piece. Luckily, in high school, the Raucher's house was one I practically lived at, so her parents are like second parents to me.

Because I was the first of my family to get to where Dad was, I had a little time alone with him to try and joke around. He was in great spirits and as funny as ever. I, however, was trying hard not to cry and act like a baby.

HOW WILL HE KNOW?

As He Gets Wheeled Away . . .
What if this is goodbye?
What if he doesn't know how much he means to me?
Does he know how much he's shaped my life?
Does he know that sitting together eating breakfast before
school each day means the world to me?
Does he know that his wry sense of humor cracks me up and
is the top quality I look for when I meet a boy I like?
Have I returned that same love to him?
How will he know?

Poem by Tina, early 20s

The transplant team says to help keep everyone's spirits up and to think positive, but be real! Human nature gets the best of everyone sometimes and you have to face the reality that this is a life-threatening proposal to have such a surgery. That's why some people elect not to have their name put on the recipient list. They decide to take their chances and just live out whatever time they have left without the anxiety, worry of money, and waiting. I knew in my heart three awful words, "He might die." No one says the words out loud, but I think we were all thinking it, even if only in the back of our minds.

My dad's surgery lasted a bit longer than expected because of massive scar tissue from previous abdominal surgeries. Then they had to reopen him after they had finished and he remembers saying, "No, don't do it." It's funny that he was alert enough to protest more surgery. Naturally the surgeons ignored him and fixed what they needed to, and he was fine.

Because the surgery lasted approximately 13–15 hours, my family stayed in the waiting room the whole time. Dad says that he's always felt bad about that, but I can't imagine why. Where else on Earth could we possibly want to be? Do parents know how special and one-of-a-kind they are to us? Heck, my parents have five kids, but we only have one mom and one dad!

For the first year or so after his transplant, my dad was so weepy. He'd cry over anything even remotely sentimental, which was a bit frightening for me because I only saw him cry one other time (and he didn't know I was watching) when he got a phone call that his mother had died. But now, right after his transplant, he'd see a family photo and smile and choke back tears.

For recipients especially, it is emotional right after the transplant. It's like they've been holding it all in for so long . . . so many fears, hopes, expectations, that the release of it can take a year or more. Sometimes it can be like floodgates opening and every emotion just pours out!

Although my dad has had minor complications over the years, his overall health has been great. Normal illnesses like the flu always throw off his medication (vomiting or diarrhea pass the medications through his system too quickly and sometimes they are not absorbed properly), which causes problems. He seems to end up in the hospital for a week, every year or two, from these complications. Nothing major is ever found; he simply is told it was a medication problem. We are all so thankful that, 9 years later, he is doing well and is still here in our lives.

TEENS AND YOUNG ADULTS ARE ASKED WHAT THEY REMEMBER ABOUT FINALLY SEEING THEIR PARENTS AFTER THE OPERATION

Ann, whose mother had a double-lung transplant in 2002, got to see her mom for the first time 5 days after surgery, because she lived far from home. Ann said, "My mom looked like a ghost. She was white and looked sickly. She couldn't talk much at that point. I was just glad she had made it to that point so far. I was happy to see her face."

A young woman named Stoney, whose father had a liver transplant, said, "My dad had so many tubes in him. I was so tired. It had to be close to being 24 hours since the whole thing started and I hadn't slept. Once I did see him, I felt that things were going to be okay."

Another young lady, Lisa, whose father also had a liver transplant said, "When I finally got to see him, it was such a relief, but kind of scary. I knew he'd have a lot of tubes, but I wasn't prepared for him to be so drugged up. He was trying to rip out tubes and was in horrible pain. The big respirator tube that was down his throat so he could breathe was really annoying for him and made his throat so dry it still felt hard to breathe. My father said the tube hurt his throat for several days, even after being removed. Also, right after surgery, he was not coming out of the [anesthesia] drugs for what seemed like forever. Once he was finally truly conscious, we were all so relieved, but in the beginning it was pretty scary."

WHAT STILL ANNOYS ME

The years following my father's surgery I'd let myself get down sometimes. Many times I'd ask myself, "Do the doctors know *anything* about us?" It seems like every time my dad gets sick with something minor like a bad cold or the flu, he ends up in the hospital. Although his medical history is detailed in his chart, it is as if no one even reads the first page, especially the part about him having an organ transplant. They always start with, "What brings you here today?" It drives me crazy!

One time, my dad was hospitalized from a bad drug interaction. Very suddenly, his muscles all atrophied. (They were like rubber and didn't work.) He couldn't even crawl upstairs to his bedroom. It was almost like he was instantly paralyzed.

Important Fact: Did You Know . . . **Because of compromised immune system after transplantation (medication given to offset organ rejection), babies who have had a liquid form of live virus vaccines should not have close contact with recipient for 3–5 days. The virus can be passed on through their stool in their diapers. Exposure to a live virus could be extremely dangerous for a transplant recipient because they are on immunosuppressant drugs. To be safe, simply check with your transplant team when dealing with vaccines.**

There was a medication that caused a problem called *rhabdomylosis*, which is the medical term for rapid muscle breakdown, which occurred in some patients. In fact, during the 4 years that drug was on the market (it isn't available anymore), 31 people in the United States died from problems related to rhabdomylosis.[2]

While in the hospital during that same episode, dad was given pancakes and syrup. He was *so* excited! He said, "Wow, is this diabetic-friendly?" and the nurse jumped right up and said, "You're diabetic? No way, you can't have this!" I was so mad. I could see the neon "diabetic" sticker in his chart from across the room where I was sitting, so I know it was there if anyone would just glance at his chart briefly. Imagine if he had eaten syrup in his condition!

I'm sure it is very frustrating to work in the medical field right now, between the HMOs having a say on every medical recommendation the hospital gives and trying to alter doctor recommendations to cut costs whenever possible, as well as downsizing of staffs to the bare minimum. (A great example of this is the movie *John Q*, starring Denzel Washington.) That still does not excuse the fact that patients' lives are being put at risk. Human error will always be a reality in any job, and the health profession is no exception.

My dad has a huge three-ring binder that contains: his medical history, medications he's taking, history of any drug interactions/reactions or problems, any experimental drugs tested on him, and any problems with amounts and combinations or medicines that were being adjusted. It is his personal "bible," his story, and he has to bring it with him to every hospital visit or grave errors could occur.

Needing to record everything in this book, especially to keep his medications straight in the first few months, was depressing for him. It was like studying for medical school! Everyone's parent is not as organized as mine, so if your parent needs help keeping it all straight, perhaps you can suggest a binder and help organize it.

My dad *never* would have believed that some day his medication regime would be second nature to him. At first, it was so confusing and difficult. The support person (spouse, sibling, kids, parents, whomever) *really* has to help out a lot at first. Not only could your parent (or you) feel sick, but might also be a bit confused, tired, crabby, depressed, and even nauseous while doctors tweak the exact combination of drugs necessary to recover and maintain the foreign object (the new organ) like it was the recipient's own.

Remember, the transplant patient's body will continue to fight against the donated organ for the rest of its life. The body will *never* recognize the new organ as its "own." Therefore, it will always try to rid itself of that object. It is truly amazing that anyone figured out how to "trick" the brain into accepting another organ in the first place!

You'll learn that your family is the best advocate to keeping you or your parent healthy. It is always best to ask about every medication given so you can be sure there aren't any allergies or drug interactions.

TRANSPLANT GAMES

The Transplant Games are like the Olympics for people who have either had heart, liver, lung, kidney, pancreas, or bone marrow transplants. (All are life-saving transplants.) An organization called the World Transplant Games Federation oversees all the games. Each event has a local organizing committee. The games are held every 2 years at various cities.[3]

On March 20, 2003, in New York, the National Kidney Foundation invited transplant recipients, families, medical professionals, and the public to celebrate the 50th anniversary of transplantation. The festivities took place at the 2004 U.S. Transplant Games held July 27–August 1, 2004 in Minneapolis, Minnesota.

The games, presented by the National Kidney Foundation (NKF), are the largest Olympic-style sports event in the world for people who have had life-saving organ transplants. The Transplant Games have grown from 1,000 people in

***Honorary Chairman of 2004 U.S.
Transplant Games***
**Dr. Joseph E. Murray and Dr. E. Donnall
Thomas received the 1990 Nobel
Prize for Medicine for their pioneering
work in organ transplantation. In
recognition of Dr. Murray's
contributions and the 50th
anniversary of the first successful
kidney transplant, he had been named
the Honorary Chairman of the 2004
U.S. Transplant Games. Upon hearing
the news, Dr. Murray, now 84 years of
age, responded, "I look forward to
attending this wonderful celebration
as I have been a supporter of the
Transplant Games for many years."[4]**

Indianapolis in 1990 to more than 8,000 in Orlando in 2002.
The 5-day event featured recognition and educational
experiences for recipient families; families who have donated
loved ones' organs, living donors, and medical experts. To
inquire about the games, you can send an e-mail to:
transplant@kidney.org, or for more information call the Kidney
Foundation at (800) 622-9010.

In August 1999, Sean Elliott of the San Antonio Spurs (NBA
professional team) had a kidney transplant, thanks to his
brother Noel's donation. Elliott returned to pro ball only 7
months after his transplant!

Other celebrities that have taken part in the games as
participants or presenters are profiled in Chapter 11. You
go to www.transweb.org to see more details about the
games.

"U.S. HEART TRANSPLANT TEEN SNOWBOARDING HER WAY TO GOLD"

When Lacey Wood was only 18 months old a virus attacked her heart. She received the heart of a 22-month-old boy. Now 13-years-old, Lacey, who is from northern California, went to the 2002 "Transplant Winter Games" in Switzerland and Italy.

She said before going, "I know life is precious. I want to squeeze ever bit of fun out of it. . . . I can't wait to get to Europe and meet a ton of new friends from all over the world." Lacey and her mom Colleen hope to raise awareness of the crucial need for donors. Colleen said, "The next time a child needs a heart, I want to do everything in my power to make sure one is available."[5]

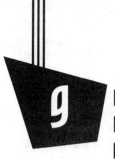

Minorities and International Patients Having Transplants

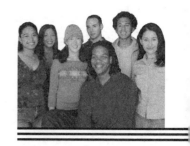

What does MOTTEP stand for?
MOTTEP is the National Minority Organ Tissue and Transplant Education Program. There are fifteen chapters around the United States.[1]

WHAT DOES THE ORGANIZATION MOTTEP DO?

National MOTTEP is the first program of its kind in the country and is designed to do the following things:

- ◎ Educate minority communities on facts about organ and tissue transplantation.
- ◎ Empower and allow minority communities to become involved in addressing the shortage of donors by developing transplant education programs.
- ◎ Increase minority participation in organ/tissue transplant services such as signing donor cards.
- ◎ Encourage and increase family discussion related to organ and tissue donation. Stress the importance of telling and retelling your loved ones of your wishes to be a donor.
- ◎ Increase the number of minorities who donate organs and tissues.[2]

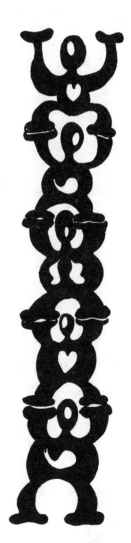

WHY IS THERE A NATIONAL MOTTEP?

"National MOTTEP® was originally established to increase the number of minority organ and tissue transplant donors. The mission of National MOTTEP® was later revised to incorporate a preventive focus by addressing the diseases and behaviors which lead to the need for transplantation such as diabetes, hypertension, alcohol and substance abuse, poor nutrition and lack of exercise."[3]

Dr. Clive O. Callender, who wanted to start an organization that would target minorities and educate them on the importance of organ donation, founded the national MOTTEP in 1991. He also wanted to encourage them to become organ donors. The idea originally began in 1978 when members of the Southeastern Organ Procurement Foundation (SEOPF) and Dr. Callender wanted to better understand why minorities, especially African Americans, had less than a 5% donation rate. The donor numbers were not in proportion to their needs. Their rate of end-stage renal disease (ESRD) was huge at the time. African Americans represented 50–70% of the dialysis population!

With a $500 grant from Howard University Hospital, Dr. Callender started a pilot project to identify the reasons African Americans were not donating. Forty African American Washington, D.C., residents were interviewed over the course of 1 year. During that time, five reasons African Americans were not donating were identified. They included:

- Lack of community awareness about renal disease and transplantation
- Religious beliefs and superstitions
- Distrust of the medical community
- A fear that by signing an organ donor card, medical personnel would not work as hard to save them
- Racism—they felt that their organs would only go to whites.

Dow Chemical Company and the National Association for the Advancement of Colored People (NAACP) helped to develop donor education programs in the historically black colleges and universities and were successful in educating the population.

DIFFERENT FROM A AND B IS NASTY HEPATITIS C

The virus Hepatitis C shows up twice as much in African Americans, while the success rates in treatment isn't nearly as high.[4] The National Institutes of Health is doing research to study possible reasons for this statistic.

Side effects from current treatment of Hepatitis C can vary from mild to horrible. Things like depression, anemia, hair loss, fatigue, thyroid problems, and severe head and backaches can be some side effects. It seems there might be a need for new treatments of the disease.

HOW DISEASES AFFECT MINORITIES DIFFERENTLY

You might find the following websites helpful:
www.liverfoundation.org (American Liver Foundation)
www.illinois-liver.org (Illinois Chapter of American Liver Foundation)
www.cdc.gov/ncidod/diseases/hepatitis/index.htm (Centers for Disease Control and Prevention)
www.my.webmd.com/condition_center_hub/hep (WebMD Hepatitis Center)
www.HepatitisMag.com (Hepatitis Magazine)

Because some diseases of the kidney, heart, lung, pancreas, and liver are found more often in racial and ethnic minority groups than in general population, let's begin with a breakdown of various diseases and health issues within these groups in the United States.

African Americans

- Approximately 2.3 million African Americans have diabetes. One third of them do not know it.

- African Americans are 1.7 times more like to have diabetes, than non-Latino whites.

- 25% of African Americans between the ages of 65 and 74 have diabetes.

- One in four African American women over 55 years of age have diabetes.[5]

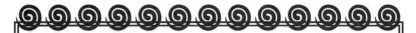

DORIAN WILSON, M.D.

Dr. Dorian Wilson is one of only 19 African American transplant surgeons. He is an assistant professor in the Department of Surgery, Division of Surgical Transplantation at the University of Medicine and Dentistry of New Jersey at the New Jersey Medical School.[6] In 1988 and 1989, he was one of the original members of the surgical team that introduced liver transplantation to University Hospital, Newark, New Jersey. He later fulfilled a commitment and was commissioned as a major in the U.S. Air Force. He performed liver, kidney, and pancreas transplants from 1993 until 1996 before returning to UMDNJ.

Native Americans

- Native Americans have the highest rates of diabetes in the world.

- Type 2 diabetes among Native Americans is 12.2% for those over 19 years of age.

- Diabetes has reached epidemic proportions among Native Americans. Complications from diabetes are major causes of death and health problems in most Native American populations.

- Amputations among Native Americans are three to four times higher than the general population.[7]

Hispanics/Latinos

- Type 2 diabetes is two times higher in Latinos than in non-Latino whites.

- 1.2 million of all Mexican Americans have diabetes.

- Nearly 16% of Cuban Americans in the United States between the ages of 45–74 have diabetes.

◎ Approximately 24% of Mexican Americans in the United States and 26% of Puerto Ricans between the ages of 45–75 have diabetes.[8]

Hypertension (also referred to as *high blood pressure*) and Minorities

◎ 23% of Americans aged 20–74 have hypertension.

◎ Over three quarters of women aged 75 and older have hypertension.

◎ 64% of men aged 75 and older have hypertension.

◎ As many as 50 million Americans age 6 and older have hypertension.

◎ Hypertension is most prevalent in the African American population. It affects about one out of every three African Americans.

◎ One in five Americans has hypertension.

◎ Non-Hispanic blacks and Mexican Americans are more likely to suffer from hypertension than are non-Hispanic whites.

◎ Over 14,000 deaths each year are attributed to hypertension.

◎ Complications include: heart attack, stroke, kidney failure, and blindness.[9]

Benefits of Regular Physical Activity

According to the Centers for Disease Control, National Center for Chronic Disease Prevention and Health Promotion, regular physical activity that is done most days of the week reduces the risk of developing, or dying from, some of the leading causes of illness and death in the United States. Regular physical activity improves health in the following ways:

◎ Reduces the risk of dying prematurely.

◎ Reduces the risk of dying from heart disease.

◎ Reduces the risk of developing diabetes.

- Reduces the risk of developing high blood pressure.
- Helps reduce blood pressure in people who already have high blood pressure.
- Helps control weight.
- Helps build and maintain healthy bones, muscles, and joints.
- Helps older adults become stronger and better able to move about without falling.[10]

Examples of Moderate, or Average, Amounts of Activity

- Washing and waxing a car for 45–60 minutes
- Playing volleyball for 45 minutes
- Playing touch football for 30–45 minutes
- Gardening for 30–45 minutes
- Walking 1 3/4 miles in 35 minutes (or 20 minutes per mile)
- Basketball (shooting baskets) for 30 minutes
- Playing a basketball game for 15–20 minutes
- Bicycling five miles in 30 minutes
- Pushing a stroller one mile in 30 minutes
- Water aerobics for 30 minutes
- Swimming laps for 20 minutes
- Jumping rope for 15 minutes
- Stair-walking for 15 minutes

(*Note from website:* To avoid soreness and injury, individuals contemplating an increase in physical activity should start out slowly and gradually build up to the desire amount to give the body time to adjust. Please consult a physician before beginning a new program of physical activity.)[1]

ORGAN DONATION

According to UNOS, as of June 2004, more than 86,000 persons were on the national transplant waiting list. Approximately 50% represent minorities:

- African Americans 23,848
- Hispanics/Latinos 12,980
- Asian/Pacific Islanders 4,527
- Other 1,944

DO HOSPITALS IN THE UNITED STATES ONLY PERFORM TRANSPLANTS ON U.S. CITIZENS?

No. Patients from other countries may travel here to receive transplants. Once accepted by a UNOS transplant center, international patients receive organs based on the same policies as U.S. citizens.

CELEBRITY RAPPER LAUNCHES DONOR RECRUITMENT CAMPAIGN

Superstar Nelly and his sister Jackie Donahue launched the "Jes Us 4 Jackie" campaign, which is a nationwide effort to bring attention to the need for marrow and blood stem cell donors. Jackie needs a marrow transplant and is searching for a donor. "The Jes Us 4 Jackie" campaign intends to bring hope not only to Jackie but also to the many patients worldwide in need of a marrow or blood stem cell donor.

Each year, more than 30,000 people are diagnosed with life-threatening diseases that can be helped or cured by a marrow or blood stem cell transplant. The campaign put together by Nelly and his sister Jackie will focus on recruiting more African American donors and donors of mixed heritage. Because tissue types are inherited, like your hair or eye color, patients are more likely to find a matching donor within their own racial or ethnic groups. That's why it is so important to increase awareness and donation rates in these various ethnic groups.

LUNG DISEASE AND MINORITIES

Although lung disease affects all people, no matter their age, gender, nationality, or race, some of the population is at higher risk for it because of living conditions. For example, people living in substandard, roach-infested housing, often in urban areas, are at higher risk.

Some minority groups are at higher risk for certain lung diseases genetically. Other factors that increase a population risk of lung disease are less access to health education and quality medical care. Research is being done to study how genetics affect varieties of lung disease.

If the trends continue to rise at the same rate they have been, research estimates that 1.6 million African Americans who are younger than 18 years old now will become regular smokers. Almost half of those people, perhaps 500,000, will end up dying of a smoking-related disease.

Because certain illnesses happen more often in different ethnic groups, pay attention to what you are at higher risk of developing. For example, if you have a higher risk of lung disease, do your best to never start smoking. Heck, don't bother to even try it! Why tempt yourself by doing something that is seriously bad for you when you may quickly and easily get hooked on it?

SEE WHO YOUR REAL FRIENDS ARE

You'll be surprised to see your real friends could care less if you do or don't do certain things, like smoke or drink. Sure, they might give you a hard time, but when it comes down to it, your real friends won't care about that stuff.

Smoking is a huge deal that the government has finally started to treat with great care. There are public service messages on TV and in print ads by celebrities. There is even more awareness by the movie industry to not glamorize smoking in films, at least not nearly as often as they did in the past. When they show smoking, it is not usually in a positive way.

Did you know Native Americans have higher-than-average smoking rates? Did you know that in the 1990s there was a substantially huge increase in the number of African Americans who started smoking? You can get addicted to it very quickly, so don't bother to even try it! If you just think of the serious cash you'll blow, yikes! *"Fah-geht-about-it!"*

ASTHMA AND MINORITIES AND TEENS

The rate of asthma among Puerto Rican children has been shown to be higher than any other Hispanic group. Puerto Ricans with asthma have also been found to have lower lung function, higher risk of emergency room visits, and longer duration of asthma than other Hispanics. Blacks are three times as likely to be hospitalized for asthma treatment than white children.[12]

JESICA SANTILLAN: A PERSONAL STORY TURNS TRAGIC

Jesica Santillan was a 17-year-old Mexican girl, illegally smuggled into the United States and moved to the Durham, North Carolina, area because of Duke University Hospital's great reputation in the transplant community.[13]

A horrible tragedy ensued when a medical error of noncompatible blood types caused Jesica to need a *second* set of heart/lungs, but it was too late. The error ultimately killed her.

The Santillan family was lucky to have twice found matching organs of rare combinations of lungs and a heart. It was almost like winning a lottery with odds of a zillion-to-one.

Even without the error that ultimately caused her death, Jesica's prognosis was grave at best. It was a long shot that may have ended similarly, days later, had the error not occurred.

The public was outraged by the fact that Jesica was brought here illegally and given two sets of lungs and two hearts, especially with the prognosis for her survival incredibly low. What people may not realize is that a percentage of donors are not U.S. citizens, so in fairness, the recipient list does not limit those getting transplants to U.S. citizens.

To fuel the fire of the public's rage, after Jesica died, her family did not donate her organs. (Even I was upset when first hearing the story, but like all stories, I know there are always two sides to be explored.) As it turned out, none of her organs were viable (or able to be used) because of medication used to save her life; plus some organs were needed for the autopsy to verify exactly what killed Jesica. That fact was never widely publicized, just reported on after the hysteria died down.

The loss of young life was catastrophic on so many levels. Human error, Jesica's death, and six other potential recipients passed up for transplantation adds up to a story of total sadness.

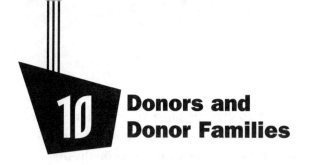

10 Donors and Donor Families

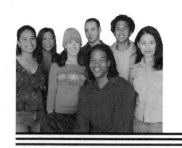

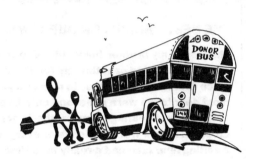

> **Simply Say Thanks**
> A source at UNOS says, "[they]
> would encourage all transplant
> recipients to remember the best
> way to thank your donor family
> is the simplest way: Just Say
> Thanks! Send a card or letter
> saying how grateful you are and
> what the transplant has meant
> to your life and your family. . . .
> You could help them as much as
> they have helped you."

TO WRITE A LETTER OR NOT TO WRITE A LETTER (TO THE DONOR FAMILY)

When I had my first child, I wrote a thank you letter to the donor family. It was less than a year after my dad's transplant surgery. I wanted the members to know how significant their gift was to me *personally*. Because I'm the youngest kid out of five, I felt very angry and cheated before my father's surgery that my siblings were all married and had kids who knew my father. I wasn't even married, let alone having any kids who would ever meet or remember their grandpa!

For our donor family to give me more time with my father was an amazing gift that cannot be expressed with words. But I still felt compelled to try. I only hope it brought the family members comfort and not more grief or anger over their loss.

Dad said he wrote to the family, too. Some of my siblings did as well, but none of us have ever received a response. Although receiving letters might be a comfort to some, I imagine responding to them can be too emotional for others.

THE BEST CHOICE FOR OUR FAMILY

The loss of my brother Juan's life, due to an accident, was the most excruciating pain that my family and I had gone through since first losing my father to cancer a year earlier. Two people most dear to me were gone, and only 1 year apart.

When first hearing of my brother's accident, my heart dropped. I knew from the looks of everyone, my father was awaiting him. Juan had a really hard time with our father's death. Who could have imagined he would be reunited with him so quickly? Juan was always trying to be a better person and was working hard for his wife and children, only to have all of our lives changed by his fatal accident.

While Juan lay in his hospital bed, Mom and I knew that he would not be walking out of there. Trauma to his head, he wasn't even conscious. At the hospital, Sam Oliveras with the California Transplant Donor Network (CTDN) came to my mother, my sister-in-law, and me with options. It was inevitable that my brother was passing on. We sat with Sam and there wasn't any question about what to do. Juan was an extremely giving person and we loved the opportunity for him to not only save the lives of others in need of organs, but felt he would live on through other people. No one can replace a loved one, or the memories of him, but meeting Crystal Capser and Ted Z., two of the three of Juan's recipients, was the greatest gift. My brother is living on. Keeping in close contact with Crystal, as she has become an active member of my family, makes us all glad we made the decision of "Gift of Life"! We cannot take the pain away of our loss, but we gained an addition to our family.

Love always, Trina Lozano

I cannot even imagine being approached at the moment you find out a family member is clinically dead; and then have to put emotions aside to decide if donating tissues and/or organs of your family member to help save other lives is what your loved one would have wanted. Because of the crucial time crunch involved, it is not possible for hospitals to give the family any time to grieve, let alone catch their breath. Every moment counts. I have the largest amount of respect for a family

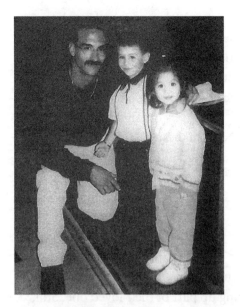

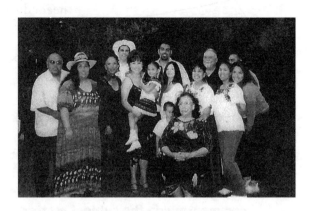

Donor Juan Namowicz with children Issac and Lorena; Crystal Capsar, kidney/pancreas recipient (holding Lorena) with her donor's family August 2003

that, during its greatest tragedy, can be generous enough to give the gift of hope to another family.

Not every family has discussed the topic of organ donation, especially if the person who is dying is very young. That is why I stress and restress the importance of sharing your wishes with your family about being an organ donor. If that decision ever has to be made, your family should not have to struggle with the decision. Relatives should just know immediately what you wanted.

Be sure to tell your family you want to be a donor, and then tell them again. It's like a TV commercial. An advertiser knows best that to make enough of an impact for you to even vaguely remember the product, each potential customer must see the ad at *least* three times. Ever notice how radio ads all mention their

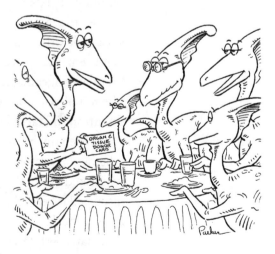

DONORSAURS

DISCUSS THEIR DECISIONS WITH FAMILY MEMBERS

143

phone number at least three times? It's a proven fact that three is the minimum number of times seeing or hearing needed to make an impression on a person. Although every major religion worldwide has publicly stated that it considers organ donation the highest form of humanitarianism, some families still struggle with religious beliefs they fear might conflict with donating organs. Yet others are just uncertain about their own feelings on giving up part of their loved one. Still, many people make that choice to donate.

Religious Groups' Views on Organ Donation
If you go to the website by the California Transplant Donor Network (www.CTDN.org) you can access specific statements from every major religion on their views of transplantation, donation, and also see commentary on the subject matter.

ILLINOIS SECRETARY OF STATE MAKES GREAT STRIDES FOR ORGAN DONATION

Jesse White was elected the 37th Illinois Secretary of State in November 1998. In November 2002, he was reelected by winning all 102 counties and receiving more than 2.3 million votes—the largest vote total by any candidate for Illinois statewide office in a quarter of a century. Although his list of achievements in programs to help underprivileged youths, literacy programs, and tougher DUI laws is unbelievable, I'd like to tell you about how he helped the cause for organ donation. It started in 1981 when Jesse's brother George died.[1]

"When my brother passed away, we had never talked about whether he wanted to be an organ donor," White said. "When I was asked about donating his organs, I said no. Maybe if we had discussed it beforehand, and there was more information available at the time, his organs could have provided life for others." Ten years later, White's sister Doris received a kidney transplant, making White a true believer and advocate of the program.

Although Illinois has the largest donor registry nationwide now, thanks to Jesse White's efforts, there are still more than

5,000 people in Illinois alone waiting for a transplant. More than 300 people in the state died the previous year, while waiting on the transplant list.[2]

In 2001, special Organ Donor License Plates were made honoring the late Chicago Bears great Walter Payton. It was made to raise public awareness of the crucial need for organ and tissue donors, featuring the Chicago Bears' navy blue and orange colors with Payton's number 34 and the familiar organ donor "Life Goes On" symbol.

DEBATE OVER DONOR ANONYMITY

Crystal Capser, a kidney/pancreas recipient, says that the system set up now with anonymity between donors and recipients is similar to the old-fashioned "closed adoption" policies. It might be necessary in the beginning weeks after surgery, but if both parties want to seek each other out, then the organization that linked them up should go that extra step to help them get in touch. Luckily, after time, she was put in touch with her donor's family, the Namowiczes. Crystal shares an amazing story of her relationship with her donor family, along with a photograph, in Chapter 5.

Gift of Hope says, "Initially letters to and from donor families will not contain last names, addresses and other information that might identify you or the donor family to each other. Gift of Hope (in Illinois) and your transplant center will release your name and address to your donor family only when you and they have both agreed to do so."[3] Each state has different policies. Crystal Capser lives in California.

Every donor family I have ever spoken to personally said that their loved one was shown the utmost care and respect. They had made the right choice and felt comfort in their decision to help the circle of life go on. Families must do what's best for them and what is within their comfort zone. You have to believe in the doctors and the Hippocratic Oath they took to "do no harm." Know that your family member is their first priority. It is absolutely the case for organ donation.

The point is not to end one life to save another. Once all avenues are exhausted and the potential donor is in fact dead, then a transplant team will use whatever viable (or usable) organs or tissues the family has allowed to be donated to help others in need.

THE CONTROVERSY OF DONOR INCENTIVES

In June 2002, the Organ Procurement and Transplantation Network (OPTN) and United Network for Organ Sharing (UNOS) board of directors agreed to allow studies of the impact of incentives to encourage organ donation and honor organ donors, then monitor their outcomes.[4]

Because volunteers are the basic foundation of public policy regarding organ donation, that idea has some people upset. The problem is there is a growing organ shortage and to do a study in a sensitive manner before the shortage is catastrophic seemed like the best solution for now.

Some potential incentives discussed include a "medal of honor" to be presented to donor families, possible reimbursement of donor funeral or medical expenses, or perhaps charitable contributions on the donor's behalf. It would not include any monetary or other "valuable consideration" in return for organ donation. That would be a direct violation of the National Organ Transplant Act, a federal law.

THE FOUNDATION FOR DONOR AND FAMILY FUNDS ASSISTANCE

The Foundation Donor and Family Funds Assistance started when a man named Judson S. Weekly donated a kidney to his mother. She had been on dialysis for quite some time and was finally eligible for a kidney transplant. Through testing, they discovered her son was two points away from being a perfect match for her![5]

At first, she said that she would not allow one of her children to be cut up, especially on her behalf. But Judd was relentless and after reading any research he could get his hands on by other donors and recipients who had gone through the procedure, and studying the statistics of outcomes, he was able to educate himself thoroughly about the process. He went back to his mother telling her what he learned and was able to convince her, as he says, "to allow me the honor of donating one of my kidneys to her." He began working with the transplant team immediately.

The year 2001 marked the first time ever in transplant history that more organs were used from live donors, such as a brother donating a kidney to his sister, than deceased donors, 6,530 versus 6,082.[6]

Everything seemed perfect and all details under control, but there was a problem. Although the insurance company would cover the procedure and the medications needed afterward, there were many more expenses to consider.

Physically helping his mom with her surgery was an easy decision for Judd, even though she lived in Arizona, and he lived in North Carolina with his wife and three kids. For the family to fly to Arizona and live there for at least a month (over Christmas and the millennium New Year) would be quite expensive. With food, hotel, airfare, car rental, and so forth, they figured it would cost approximately $6,000. Fortunately, a family member donated his frequent flier miles to Judd so he could get to Arizona for the surgery. Because it would take place around the winter holidays, Judd worried about being without his wife and kids for the holidays, and during the possible dangers of the Y2K changeover that were so hyped.

The strain that could keep the family apart during the transplant was related to some financial troubles caused by a few unforeseen tragedies, including a fire and theft, and the family's entire savings account was pretty much wiped out.

That's when they found out that Judd's mom was finally eligible for a kidney transplant. The stress of the situation was almost too much for Judd and Jennifer to bear. But Judd's mother had been a slave to the dialysis machine (needed to clean her blood, because her kidneys couldn't do the job) for so long that he knew a transplant would ultimately be the answer to everyone's prayers.

Because Judd's mother had to go to dialysis several hours a week, it ruined her chances of advancement at work. Judd was often frustrated by this and wanted his mom to be freed of the burden of her illness forever!

A TV station heard about Judd's and his mother's situation and wanted to do a local story. After discussing it, Judd and Jennifer decided it made them too uncomfortable. They didn't want to appear as though they were begging for money. They were used to being the ones helping people, not asking for handouts.

When a local newspaper heard of their predicament, too, they offered to do an article. This they could agree to and were happy to accept the offer of a newspaper article. After a quick interview and a 5-minute photo session of the family, the story seemed pretty low profile and elegant.

Much to their surprise, the Saturday that the story ran, Judd and Jennifer's phone began ringing at 9:00 A.M. and didn't stop for days. People called to share well wishes, prayers, and offers of monetary support as well. Even local businesses called willing to pay for Jennifer and the kids' plane fares.

Then a local radio station got wind of the story and started promoting it too. Soon, there was $20,000 in donations for the family! They decided with all this goodwill they were receiving, no family should be in this predicament ever again. They decided to use as much of the funds that they could spare to start the Foundation for Donor and Family Funds Assistance. They say they plan to make their efforts global in scope and believe that all men and women are created equal, regardless of their nationality or birthplace. This foundation is set up to help as many families of living donors as possible.

BETH BOWERS: A DONOR'S STORY

In 2002, a young woman named Elizabeth Rachel Bowers became an organ donor. At the time of her death, she was a healthy, 22-year-old woman working in the Peace Corps in Zambia, Africa. She graduated as valedictorian of her class from Sprague High School, Salem, Oregon, in 1997 and had been a cheerleader, a choir member, a pianist, and held a black belt in karate. She went on to graduate Phi Beta Kappa from Earlham College in Richmond, Indiana. Originally, Beth wanted to study to become part of the FBI but ended up choosing Earlham because of the Quaker school's peace and global studies program.

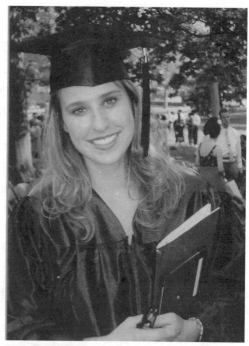

Elizabeth Rachel Bowers—organ donor

Beth could have gone to an Ivy League college like her parents, who are both English professors at Willamette University. But she chose a less popular path of service, being the individual that she was. In college, she took up snowboarding, skydiving, and continued her horseback riding. She wanted to enlarge her perspective of the world and her place in it. Therefore, she spent her junior year at Waseda University in Japan before returning to Earlham. She graduated in 2001 with a major in Japanese studies. She went to Zambia in early September 2001.

Her parents supported her wishes to join the Peace Corps and spent 2 months with her before she left for Zambia. This helped them emotionally prepare themselves to let her go to Africa. Linda Bowers said her daughter was driven by a desire to give back to the world because she had such a loving, privileged upbringing. "You don't come between a person and her dream, a person and her destiny," Linda said. Her daughter had a spiritual quality that set her apart. She was easygoing, direct, and self-assured. She loved adventure and was not afraid of the unknown.

Beth agreed to serve in Zambia for 2 years. Poverty was apparent all around her. One more thing that would have singled her out as being one of the privileged ones was her Peace Corps–issued bike helmet. She was compassionate and sensitive to others around her and didn't want to draw attention to the economic differences. However, if she had been wearing her bike helmet, her life might have been spared.

On February 25, 2002, Beth was biking down a hill when she hit something on the road and fell. A priest found her and rushed her to a local hospital. When the doctors realized her head injury was serious, she was airlifted to South Africa. For a while it seemed as if she would recover, but 4 days after doctors operated, she got an infection and swelling of the brain. She was then put on life support.

After speaking with Beth's mother, Linda, I learned that the Peace Corps had originally called her with vague information. They could only tell her that there was an accident and Beth had sustained severe head trauma. Because it would be a 2-day trip to get to her, Beth's parents decided to have one person stay in the states to remain in contact with the hospital. When Gerry arrived in Pretoria, "The Peace Corps was there for support every minute and was usually three steps ahead of us," Linda Bowers told me. "They were very helpful, really extraordinary."

Frances Kinghorn, an Earlham College alumna, ended up sitting with Beth until Gerry, Beth's dad, got there. Frances answered the World Wide Web call to Earlham alumnus for a civilian advocate in South Africa. She wrote e-mails to Linda to give her daily updates and was very maternal toward Beth.

Hundreds of people responded to the call for help, from Japan to Australia, India to Slovakia, and from Africa. There were prayer circles by many who didn't even know the Bowers. Gerry said he really felt a healing and supportive energy in the hospital. He also said the equipment used at the hospital was state of the art. Everything that could be done to help Beth was indeed done.

After there was no hope of Beth's survival, the family donated her usable organs and tissues. Her mother, Linda, said,

"One really hard part was that they couldn't use her heart or liver (two life saving organs) due to the medication she was given to try to save her life." But they were able to use her heart valves, and the other organs and tissues were used to save or enhance 22 South African lives!

Beth left behind parents Linda and Gerry, and her sister Jennifer. Her best friend, Berkeley Williams said, "Beth threw herself into life and managed to live more during her 22 years than most people do in a lifetime." She called Beth brilliant, a natural athlete, and the most sincere person she's ever known. "I will miss her laugh. She was always so happy. It was really infectious."

Jeani Bragg, Beth's supervisor and mentor at Tokyo International University of America (TIUA) for two summers commented, "People were drawn to her because she was friendly and thoughtful." That thoughtful spirit was apparent when, as her parents said, "There was never any question about Beth being an organ donor. It was something she had made clear, if anything had ever happened to her."

Tony Award–winning actor Mandy Patinkin, who you might know from movies or TV, received a cornea transplant in each eye.[8]

WHAT SHE DONATED

Of those people who are diagnosed "legally blind," 20,000 individuals' eyesight can be saved with cornea transplants. Both of Beth's corneas were used, and the family received handwritten anonymous letters of gratitude from both cornea recipients. One 17-year-old boy can see now, because of Beth's gift, and has returned to school.

Her kidneys helped one man and one woman to get off dialysis, allowing room for more patients to be able to get on dialysis, a gift of hope that essentially helped four people. Beth's bone tissues helped 16 people, including infants, mostly with bone cancer and tumors.

Shown Great Respect, Even in Death

When I asked Linda Bowers if the proper respect was shown to her daughter and that the family's feelings were taken into consideration by the procurement team (who usually approaches the donor family, but whom the Bowers contacted themselves immediately) she said, "Yes, absolutely."

There were messages and e-mails from all over the world to help give support to the Bowers family. Although their experience was an unimaginable tragedy, they were still able to think of others and how to make some good come out of their impossible situation. In fact, in South Africa, police had to investigate Beth's death to rule out any foul play. If there were even a chance of someone causing Beth's accident, the government would not allow her to be an organ donor. This discourages people from committing murder or "accidental deaths" to get more organs on the black market.

The nature of Beth's gift of life was extraordinary, especially because she was a stranger in a foreign land. Her thoughtfulness must surely have increased the organ donor rate in South Africa.

BRAIN AND TISSUE DONATION HELPS TO FIND CURES FOR DISEASES

Research on brain tissue has uncovered important information on developmental disorders and disabilities. Because of donations to the Brain and Tissue Banks for Developmental Disorders, advances can be made to help treat and eventually, it hopes, cure diseases.

Due to the Elizabeth Bowers' Memorial Scholarship Fund, 41 Zambian young women are now in school. For details on how to contribute to the fund, go to www.tinaPschwartz.com.

When a 3-year-old child with Rett syndrome died, her parents donated tissue from her brain for research. With the donation of that single brain, researchers have gained valuable insight into Rett syndrome, a neurological disease found only in girls. Girls with this disability develop severe dementia and autistic-like behavior as well as lose purposeful movement in the hands.[9]

The National Institute of Child Health and Development (NICHD) funds two brain and tissue banks to provide human tissues to allow investigators to study children's diseases that alter normal development or maturation of the nervous system. In 1993, the brain and tissue bank at the University of Miami School of Medicine was established. In 1996, a group bank at Children's Hospital of Orange County, California, was added, and then in 2001 it moved to Eastern Maine Medical Center in Bangor, Maine. A second NICHD-funded brain and tissue bank was established in 1991 at the University of Maryland.[10]

The diseases studied at the brain and tissue banks include autism, diseases causing mental retardation, chromosomal abnormalities, including Down's syndrome; musculoskeletal disorders like muscular dystrophy and spinomuscular atrophy, plus acquired diseases like perinatal asphyxia, and trauma. Most of the cases studied are from tissue samples taken from babies and children who died with these disorders. But the bank does collect and distribute cases (anonymous patient files) affecting adults that are similar to childhood disorders, such as ALS (amyotropic lateral sclerosis, Lou Gehrig's disease) to study for research.

As you can see, organ and tissue donation (which includes brain tissue) is used to help enhance lives, not just save people who are dying. This research will hopefully wipe out some horrific diseases in the not-so-distant future. What a generous gift to donate!

NICHOLAS GREEN: A DONOR WHO STARTED A WORLD WIDE AWARENESS OF THE POWER OF ORGAN DONATION

On September 29, 1994, the Green family (parents Reg and Maggie and 4-year-old Eleanor, and 7-year-old Nicholas) from California, was driving along the main road south from Naples while vacationing in Italy. It was at night, though not late, when a car with two men inside, faces hidden by black handkerchiefs, drove alongside the Green's car and shouted at them to stop. When the father tried to outrun them, they fired several shots at the car. In the end, the Greens did outrun their assailants and raced through the night until they saw a police car at the scene of an accident. It wasn't until they stopped that they both realized Nicholas wasn't sleeping. He had been hit in the head by a bullet and lay perfectly still. "My feeling was of senseless wastefulness," said Reg Green.

Italy was horrified by the crime, then amazed at what the Green family did in return. Rather than harbor a bitter hatred toward a country not their own, they did the most selfless act and decided to donate their son's organs to seven Italians. British-born Reg Green said of the gift, "It wasn't an issue for us. It was so obvious."[11]

Though Reg and Maggie appeared to have unwavering courage and strength, they were absolutely devastated. Their son was curious, imaginative, and intelligent. He once told his dad, "I want to know everything!" After his death, his little sister seemed to think of Nicholas as a guardian angel. Their mother Maggie tries not to think of him as an angel, "I don't want him sanitized and one-dimensional," she said. "I want to remember all his beautiful complexity."

Italy had one of the lowest rates of organ donation in Europe. The Greens' gift was one that amazed and inspired the country. Schools, parks, and streets were renamed in Nicholas's honor and parades were held. Since then, Italian donation rates have tripled so that thousands of people are alive who would have died, including many children.

Reg agrees, "He was a good boy, but he was a boy. His room was a mess, he got mad at his sister, and he was one of the most finicky eaters I've ever met." Yet the truest memories are the most painful, Reg says.

Because their story had touched so many hearts and their phone was constantly ringing off the hook with invitations to come speak and write on the subject of organ donation, they realized that this could become their life's work. In the 10 years since Nicholas's death, Reg and Maggie have written innumerable magazine articles about the shortage of organs. They have made half a dozen videotapes that are shown in hospitals, schools, and churches across the United States, which can be ordered through the producer, Corporate Productions (818/303-2622) or Richard@ CPIVIDEO.com. The Green's website is www. NicholasGreen.org.[12]

Since the video's release, it has been translated into Spanish and Italian, and there is now a second video called *Thank you, Nicholas*, which concentrates on the recipients. Its running time is 8 minutes. The cost of both videos together is approximately $12.95 U.S. dollars and can be ordered from Corporate Productions Inc., 4516 Mariots Avenue, Toluca Lake, CA 91602.

The Greens also told their story on many television shows and spoke to large audiences in both America and Europe. Reg said, "We know it is having an effect because the only sound you hear is falling tears." When they appeared on French TV, 40,000 people offered to pass on their organs when they died."

THOSE WHO NICHOLAS GREEN HELPED

When 7-year-old Nicholas Green was killed while vacationing in Italy with his family, his parents donated his organs and tissues. The seven recipients are like many others who need a transplant: a mother who had never seen her baby's face clearly; a diabetic who had been repeatedly in comas; a boy of 15 who had been wasting away with a heart disease and was only the size of a 7-year-old; a sportsman whose vision had been gradually darkening; and two children who had been hooked up to dialysis machines 3 hours a day, 4 days a week. Then there was Maria Pia, a vivacious 19-year old girl who, on the night Nicholas was shot, had been dying, too. Now against all odds, Maria Pia is in excellent health. She is married and had a baby boy in 1998, whom she named Nicholas, and she later had a baby girl.

"Few potential donors realize . . . by one action they can save other families from the devastation they themselves face. Sometimes I wonder how there can be any other choice," said Nicholas's father.

Regarding his own son's death, Reg said, "Maggie and I both thought someone should have the future he lost."[13]

OFFERING THE OPTION CAN HELP A FAMILY DEAL WITH THE LOSS OF A LOVED ONE

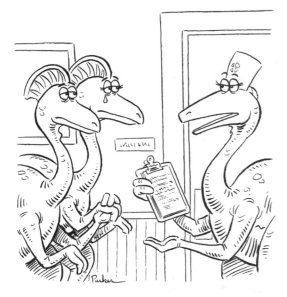

In addition, Reg and Maggie Green set up a foundation that supports UNICEF (United Nations Children's Fund) and one that gives scholarships to gifted children. "Activity helps us get through the grief," Reg said. He also said he is an agnostic, but feels close to Nicholas at the gravesite. "I sit on the bench and look at his face on the tombstone. . . . I tell him how much I miss him and as I'm leaving, I tell him when I'm coming back again." For Maggie, she finds consolation in religion. Although she was raised Presbyterian, she prays like a Roman Catholic using a rosary someone gave her in Italy. Maggie said she believes in the afterlife, "I have faith that Nicholas is out there somewhere. He has a spirit well-suited to heaven."

After being in a family who got *many* extra years with a loved one that definitely would not have happened without the transplant, I know firsthand the indescribable gratitude one feels. There is no law in place that requires potential recipients to be donors, should they die. However, why would that even need to be discussed? Wouldn't it naturally be a "given"? How can someone be willing to accept such a *rare* gift as an organ or multiple organs without being willing to do the same for others in the same position?

TOO RADICAL AN IDEA?

Perhaps a requirement to sign a donor card should be made a prerequisite to be on the organ transplant waiting list. It would certainly open up the list of available organs. There is a question of ethics to think about.

While looking at an article in *Chicago Parent* published in September 2002, a third-year medical school resident read an article about a woman named Janice. Janice was a local Chicago mother waiting for a liver transplant. The med-student was studying to be an emergency room physician and knew she would end up working with families of possible donors in her ER work. She asked Janice for a copy of the article because she wanted to be able to share it with potential donor families. She felt Janice put a human face on the issue of organ donation.

> **Gift of Hope Organ and Tissue Donor Network covers all costs related to procurement of organs in Illinois. The family only pays funeral costs.[14]**

NATIONAL DONOR RECOGNITION CEREMONY AND WORKSHOP

On July 12–13, 2003, the 8th National Donor Recognition Ceremony and Workshop was held in Washington, D.C. Donors and donor family members attended workshops and sharing sessions on Saturday. Transplant recipients and the public were invited to join them at the Sunday ceremony. There was no cost, but attendees had to preregister for the programs. They were able to download registration materials straight off the website. If you'd like information on the event, or to find out about the yearly plans, call the National Donor Family Council at 1-800-622-9010.

11 Transplant Myths, Media Coverage, and Controversies

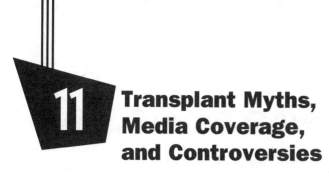

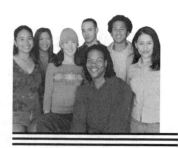

TOP 10 MYTHS ABOUT ORGAN DONATION

Myth 1: *Wealthy people and celebrities are moved to the top of the list faster than "regular" people.*

Fact: As you now know, after reading this book, that is not true. Who gets the next transplanted organ depends on factors such as matching blood and tissue types, length of time on the waiting list, how sick the person is, and how long they've been waiting on the list, not to mention how far they are located from the available organ (plus several other medical factors).

Myth 2: *Donation will mutilate my body.*

Fact: Donated organs are removed surgically, in a routine operation similar to having your appendix removed. So, for example, if you wanted an open-casket funeral, it would still be possible.

Myth 3: *My family will be charged for the surgery to donate my organs.*

Fact: Donation costs nothing to the donor's family or estate.

Myth 4: *If I'm in an accident and the hospital sees that I want to be a donor, the doctors will not try as hard to save my life.*

Fact: Organ and tissue recovery takes place only after *all* medical efforts to save your life have been exhausted and death has legally been declared. The doctors who work on you are different from the organization that asks/sees if a person wants to be a donor. That is called the OPO, or organ procurement organization. Plus, they don't get called until you are declared dead. Once the OPO is called, if and *only* if your family agrees to let you be a donor, then the transplant team is called.

(continued)

TOP 10 MYTHS ABOUT ORGAN DONATION *(CONTINUED)*

Myth 5: *I am not the right age to donate.*

Fact: You can be an organ donor from birth through almost any age. The limit for tissue donors is birth through approximately 70 years old. More of a factor than age is how well your body worked prior to death. If any organs are usable, the medical professionals will be able to determine that by factors other than how old you were.

Myth 6: *My religion does not support donation.*

Fact: All mainstream organized religions approve of organ and tissue donation and consider it an act of charity. In fact, most have publicly stated that organ donation is the "highest form of humanitarianism."

Myth 7: *Only heart, liver, and kidneys can be transplanted.*

Fact: Organs that are most needed and can be donated are: heart, kidneys, pancreas, lungs, liver, and intestines. Tissues that can be donated include the eyes, skin, bone, heart valves, and tendons.

Myth 8: *I have a history of medical illness. You would not want my organs or tissues.*

Fact: At the time of death, the medical professionals would review your medical and social histories to determine whether or not you can be a donor. With recent advances in transplantation, many more people than ever before can be donors. It's best to sign a donor card and tell your family your wishes. The appropriate officials will determine if any of your organs or tissues are usable.

Myth 9: *In my will, I have it documented that I want to be a donor, so my family doesn't need to know or even have a say in that decision.*

Fact: By the time your will is read, it will be too late to use your organs. Telling your family you want to be an organ and tissue donor now, while you are still living, is the best way to be sure your wishes are carried out. Although organ transplantation laws and technology are changing on a daily basis, as of this printing, permission must still be obtained from next of kin before any organs can be used.

Myth 10: *I heard about this fraternity guy that was drugged, then woke up to find his abdomen packed with ice. He was missing a kidney and found out it was stolen and sold on the black market!*

Fact: This is what's called an urban legend. It means it's like a "campfire story" or "ghost story" that gets told and retold with different details, like "my cousin's girlfriend's neighbor really had this happen to his brother!" when in fact, it is not a true story at all. It's been told over and over again through the years just to scare people, and people always swear, "No it's true. I know a guy who knows who it really happened to!"[1]

THE GREAT DEBATE: THE PROS AND CONS OF SELLING HUMAN ORGANS

There is an ongoing debate about whether or not to allow people to sell organs in the United States. Although the American Medical Association (AMA) has only agreed to do a study on possibly compensating families for organ donation, it will be a long time before any decisions will be made.

In 1984, Congress banned financial incentives for organ donors. There are two sides of the debate over monetary rewards for organ donors. One side suggests that if there is a price put on donating, those who are doing it out of the goodness of their heart will retreat and not donate if it becomes a "money issue."

Another point is that some fear incentives could exploit those who are poverty stricken. Naturally, the people most eager to donate will be those desperate for money. They might be people who are not in the best of health, most likely poverty stricken, without proper medical care, not to mention lacking sufficient nutrition, rendering them less healthy and attractive candidates for such a large procedure as donating an organ.

In an article in the October 8, 2002, *New York Times*, titled "When People Sell Their Kidneys," it was reported what happened in Chennai, India. The desperately poor people each donated a kidney in hopes of getting out of debt. What happened in return was their income had actually gotten smaller because of deteriorating health. Of the 305 donors interviewed in February 2001, the average money each donor was given ranged from $450 to $6,280, although most were promised much larger sums. According to the study, the average amount received was $1,070.

Considering they had to be out of work (while sick and recuperating) and not really receiving the exact money promised, the donors really got a raw deal. What's to prevent that from finally happening here in the States?

CUTTING EDGE TECHNOLOGY: DOMINO TRANSPLANTS

There is a procedure called a "domino" liver transplant. It is controversial because of the risks posed to all three patients involved.

The first risk was to the living donor, a man named Doug Andrews, who was a 32-year-old pastor. Andrews gave Jeff Cross a piece of his liver. This also represents the first controversy, "live-liver donors" and the risk to them. We'll call it "Risk #1" because it puts a healthy person into a position of undergoing an intricate, invasive, and dangerous surgery with no benefits to one's self. Doug Andrews didn't even know Jeff Cross, the man with a rare liver disease that desperately needed a transplant, but his wife had been friends with Cross since childhood.

One hurdle for Jeff Cross to overcome was finding a donor who also had "O positive" blood. As mentioned earlier in the book, even though "O" blood types are universal donors, they can only receive the exact blood type that they have. When Doug Andrews was tested and matched, after much thought, discussion, and prayer, he and his wife decided to go ahead with the donation.

After Cross got the new healthy partial liver, his diseased liver was taken out and then transplanted into a woman who had liver cancer and would have died within a year without the new organ. Risk #2 was to Mr. Cross. His heart was in bad shape and it was uncertain if he could withstand the surgery. Luckily, he came through just fine.

Last was risk #3 to the other recipient, a single mother named Lily Cheng, who had liver cancer. The biggest risk she faced was what would happen if, once in the operating room, they discovered the cancer had spread past the liver to other parts of her body. Miraculously, once in surgery, doctors discovered the cancer was contained, so they went ahead with the transplant.

Considering the complications that could have occurred in any of the three people being operated on, the surgeries all went like clockwork, relatively free of complications. There were some postoperative problems, but all were overcome relatively easily. All three patients, Cheng, Andrews, and Cross are alive and well today, thanks to the generosity of Doug Andrews.[2]

CONTROVERSIAL TOPICS

Voice Box Transplant

In a given year roughly 10,000 Americans will be diagnosed with laryngeal cancer and about 4,000 will die of the disease,

OVARY TRANSPLANT—APRIL 2004

In an Associated Press article, 24-year-old (American) identical twins took part in a rare operation. When one twin could not get pregnant, her sister, who has three daughters, donated an ovary. Doctors expect the receiving twin to begin menstruating in 3 months and hope she becomes pregnant naturally. She had tried in vitro fertilization two times, without success. It is believed that this is the first time anyone in the United States has tried such a transplant. However, China reported a successful ovary transplant between sisters in 2003.[3]

according to the American Cancer Society. In 1998 a man named Tim Heidler received the world's first voice box transplant and 3 years later was reported as physically saying, "[he] was fine."[4]

Mr. Heidler's had been in a motorcycle accident in the late 1970s that crushed his voice box and pharynx, leaving him unable to speak. He had the transplant years later, when he was 40 years old. His voice has a nearly normal quality now and he is a motivational speaker. The process used on him is described in the May 31, 2001, issue of the *New England Journal of Medicine*.

Candidates for such a procedure would include people who have suffered severe voice box trauma, destructive infections, or benign tumors. People who have had malignant masses of the larynx would also be candidates, as long as they have stayed cancer-free for at least 5 years. The surgery has not been repeated yet because the candidates for the surgery are the wrong people to be on immunosuppression therapy.

Suppressing, or slowing down, the immune system is necessary to prevent rejection of the transplanted tissues; but a weakened immune system will allow for a reoccurrence of cancer. Plus, the throat environment is prone to infection. That makes it kind of a no-win situation.

The fact that the Cleveland Clinic was successful gives great hope to people who have had their larynx removed. Although it is still in the early stages, this is a procedure to keep watching.

WHEN LIVING DONORS DIE

The December 5, 2002, episode of *60 Minutes II* profiled Vickie Hurewitz, whose husband, Mike, died after giving part of his liver to his brother. The controversy isn't over her husband's death; it is over a particular procedure that essentially was a success, but ultimately failed due to lack of aftercare provided.[6]

Because thousands of people in the United States die each year while waiting for organ transplants that will never take place due to the shortage of available organs, people sometimes

WOMB TRANSPLANT SUCCESSFUL IN RESEARCH MICE

According to a July 1, 2003, Associated Press story, Swedish scientists in Madrid, Spain, were successful in transplanting a functioning uterus into mice. In experiments, offspring were grown in the womb, and the growth and fertility of the second generation was normal. In 2002, Saudi scientists reported the first human womb transplant, which produced two menstrual periods before it failed and had to be removed. It is estimated that in approximately 3% of woman diagnosed as "infertile" the problem can be traced to the uterus. The problem with this kind of transplant for reproductive purposes is that in this surgery it is difficult to stop the drugs from attacking the new tissues (uterus) at the same time it is necessary to sustain the fetus. Developing fetuses need extra protection from infection to fight off possible problems such as birth defects.

Would the immunosuppressant drugs work and keep the uterus from rejecting, but ultimately cause damage to the fetus? Or would the fetus stay safe from harmful viruses, but die when the uterus is rejected? It seems far out of reach for now, but since it has been successful in mice, scientists are figuring out the details needed to transfer to humans and their success can't be too far off![5]

opt to be living donors. At least that has been an option for kidney donation for sometime, and more recently liver donation, as well. When a living donor gives part of his or her liver to a recipient, the donor is left with the smaller chunk. It is estimated that within 6 weeks, the liver will have regenerated itself to a full-grown, normal adult-sized liver. Amazing, isn't it? 6 weeks!

The controversy lies in taking a perfectly healthy individual and subjecting him or her to highly technical, uncommon, serious surgery where many complications could occur. Many dangerous complications happen after surgery. Some feel that the bigger threat is posed to the donor, not the recipient, when it comes to live donor liver transplants. Skeptics say that loved ones are pressured into donating, whether they admit it to themselves or not. A serious health risk is involved, not to mention the 1% risk of death to the donor. Would you consider such a risky procedure if you were a perfectly healthy individual? That's huge!

Brothers Mike and Adam Hurewitz always stood together. Adam, younger by 3 years, was a doctor on Long Island, New York. Mike, the "big brother," was a reporter at the *New York Post*. If there was anything Mike could do to help save his brother's life, he was going to do it, no matter what. Mike's wife, Vickie, agreed with his decision and supported him 100%.

After surgery, there was a horrible tragedy and Mike died. His aftercare was essentially left to a first-year resident, most likely sleep deprived, who was in charge of 34 patients by himself. (The resident confessed to feeling "overwhelmed.") When Mike took a turn

---

OFF THE HOOK

Because it is feared that relatives and close friends feel immense pressure to participate in living organ donation, and one third of potential donors back out, some doctors will secretly leave an "out" for the person. The physician can talk to potential donors alone during "pretesting" and come up with a reason not to accept them as a donor.

The fact is, whether people realize it or not, they *do* put pressure on relatives and friends to donate either by asking verbally or by hinting. It is not done intentionally and it creates a feeling of guilt on the part of the recipient as well.

for the worse, the resident couldn't reach a superior, Adam's wife ran down to the intensive care unit to find a doctor, but the physician in charge couldn't be located.

By the time a higher-ranking doctor, made it up to the unit and checked on Mike, he was unconscious and his lungs had filled with blood! He was dead. His wife was outraged. She said they wouldn't have considered the surgery had they known there would be essentially *no* aftercare provided; especially knowing that the aftercare is the most crucial part of the whole ordeal for a live donor liver transplant. The hospital knew that's when the most life-threatening things might occur.

After a review, Mt. Sinai Hospital said it would voluntarily suspend the operation and it was given 6 months to take corrective action. After officials investigated Mt. Sinai further, there were so many other complaints that an indefinite ban has been extended to the hospital. Vickie Hurewitz is suing the hospital for malpractice and is going a step further, hoping to suspend the operation everywhere. Although her husband's outcome was indeed tragic, many argue that banning the live donor liver transplant would cost many, many lives. Those who support the procedure say that one mistake shouldn't cost others their lives. Some worry that with the Mt. Sinai program being suspended, others potential recipients might be dying. Don't worry though; Mt. Sinai's medical cases have been referred to other hospitals.

SIBLINGS GIVING THE ULTIMATE GIFT TO EACH OTHER

The May 5, 2002, issue of the *New York Times Magazine* profiled three families where siblings either gave a kidney, or were about to give a kidney in a matter of weeks or months, to another sibling. It was very touching to read how each person felt. The article included direct quotes from each person, both the donor and the recipient, on feelings and emotions they were going through.[7] It'll make you cry to read, so I'll just describe each scenario briefly.

Family Profile 1: Jim and Andy Palacio

The Palacio brothers, Jim and Andy, had surgery February 20, 2002. Andy went to the emergency room with pains one day and was told his kidneys were failing. He needed to go on dialysis while they tried to find him a kidney. He didn't want to burden his loved ones, but family and friends quickly offered to help out. Approximately 15 people were on the list to be tested for him. But he still felt very unsure about it all.

Andy and his wife have two sons, one of whom has cerebral palsy. Most of the time, he carries his son Damien and puts him in his wheelchair. He didn't want to leave his wife alone to be responsible for everything in their boys' lives. Andy is a really large-sized man, so it would be hard to match him up physically. (Remember transplants need to be similar body build and type.)

Kidney matches go on a scale from 1 to 6 and siblings usually rank anywhere from 3 or 4 or 5 at best, with identical twins ranking 5 or 6 usually. The Palacio brothers have six other siblings, but Jim was the closest in body size to Andy. Amazingly, Andy and his brother Jim matched to a 6. It was like a miracle!

Jim described himself as the "black sheep of the family." It's an expression that means he was the one family member who always seems to be in trouble, or is usually known for not doing what the family wants or expects of them. He said that he knew it was the right thing to do. Andy's life meant more, especially because he had two kids depending on him. He didn't even need to ask Jim to donate, it was just understood, Jim said. He had finally made good, he guessed.

Family Profile 2: Albert Condry and Jere Jackson

Jere had kidney failure for 2 and a half years. She has six brothers and went to Hawaii, where five of them live, to get a sense of their feelings regarding transplant surgery without actually coming out to ask them to get tested.

Her brother Albert joked around with her on the phone and asked what she was calling for, a kidney? When she admitted yes, he said no problem. He'd get tested. It didn't occur to him until later, "What am I thinking?" It was all very scary and unreal, plus he was pretty wild and partied a lot. Did she really want a part of his trashed body? Although he was a smoker and drinker, it turns out he was still the healthy one.

Albert admitted that it took him quite a while to get comfortable with the transplant idea, but once he saw how weak his sister was, he knew he made the right decision.

Jere was afraid to have to ask any of her brothers for such an extraordinary gift, but had no choice. She was a wreck. Although all her brothers loved her, she sensed that Al had truly *wanted* to do it. She knew he was scared and would never commit to it. When they were finally scheduled to have the surgery in March, and were both on the tables with her brother sedated, surgeons stopped the procedure. Her blood creatinine levels were too low. The transplant has been postponed for approximately 10 months until her problem could be stabilized.

Now Albert has come to terms with the process and says he can hardly wait until the day it happens. He desperately wants to help his sister get well.

Family Profile 3: Dennis and Dana Branch

Dennis had already gone through the whole transplant ordeal. His brother Dana had gone through the tests and was found to be a match. Then 1 week before the surgery, a cadaver's kidney came through and they called Dennis from the transplant list. He knew the kidney wasn't as good a match as his brother's was, but was relieved that he didn't have to endanger his brother's life.

Unfortunately, his kidney only lasted 4½ years before failing, sending Dennis back to dialysis. When the opportunity for Dana to be a donor for Dennis came up again, he was happy to come forward to volunteer. Although the brothers have four other siblings, the others had various ailments that prevented them from being suitable donors.

Dana admitted that this time around he was much more comfortable in his decision. His kids were all in college now, so it wasn't as scary a prospect as when they were younger and he was needed in a much greater capacity. Plus, he knew he could still function normally with one kidney.

The surgery is scheduled soon. By the time you read this, you might be able to look up an update of these families at the *New York Times* website!

HIV AND TRANSPLANTATION

The question has been asked about human immunodeficiency virus (HIV) patients being able to get organ transplants, especially now that they are living much longer due to better treatments. People with HIV can be added to the UNOS list, but with informed consent that the immunosuppressive drugs that are used to treat organ rejection *may* pose a risk to their condition.

The drugs used on transplant recipients, the ones that trick a body into letting a new organ (or foreign matter) survive in a person's body, work because they lower the body's immune system. People with HIV already have a compromised immune system and don't necessarily want it weakened further. That is the biggest conflict when deciding whether or not to try for a transplant, if you have HIV.

In July 2004 Illinois State Representative Larry McKeon wrote a bill allowing people with HIV to donate organs to waiting recipients who are also HIV positive. Governor Rod R. Blagojevich signed the bill. Illinois has not ironed out all the details of how to safeguard these donations; but a separate organ donor pool will have to exist so there is no risk of a negative recipient getting the organ of an HIV-positive donor. Also, because there are different strains of the HIV virus, more medical research will be done to ensure the safety of such donations.8 (With laws changing daily, new ones may exist by the time you read this book. Check the Internet for the most up-to-date information.)

CONTROVERSIAL ANIMAL-HUMAN HEART TRANSPLANT OF 1964

Dr. James D. Hardy died in 2003 when he was 84 years old. He will be remembered for many medical firsts, one of which was for doing the first animal-human transplant. He had been doing transplant research since 1955 and by 1964, was ready to perform the first transplant of a human heart.

On January 23, 1964, 68-year-old patient Boyd Rush came to the hospital needing an immediate heart transplant. However, no human heart was available. The only chance of survival was an available chimpanzee heart.[9]

The surgery was approved and Dr. Hardy performed it. Although the new heart did beat on its own in the beginning, it was too small to maintain independent circulation and Mr. Rush died after 90 minutes. Dr. Hardy had been using both human and chimpanzee hearts in his research, but was severely criticized. As the University of Mississippi Medical Center's surgery chief, Dr. Hardy headed teams that did three pioneering operations: the first human lung transplant in 1963, the first animal-to-human heart transplant in 1964, and a double-lung transplant that left the heart in place, in 1987. He never talked about "being the first," but he was incredibly proud of developing techniques in the lab and extending them to humans. Through the years, he also became a hero to countless transplant patients.

SHOULD DEATH-ROW INMATES, OR ANY INCARCERATED PERSON, RECEIVE A TRANSPLANT?

On June 12, 2003, in Baton Rouge, Louisiana, the Senate Judiciary Committee approved a bill banning the use of state money for organ transplants for all people who have exhausted all appeals after a conviction for first-degree murder.[10]

By law, as of a 1976 U.S. Supreme Court ruling, prisoners have the right to equal medical care. That means, regarding organ transplants, taxpayers would have to foot the bill for an average cost of $200,000–500,000 surgeries, not to mention the almost $20,000-per-year follow-up medication costs. Back in the 1970s, transplants were not what they are today. They were rare medical miracles. Today, they are becoming daily occurrences. They are still miracles, but luckily, they are happening more and more often.

CLONED PIGS MISSING A GENE

Although cloning seems to be a hot topic in the United States, it comes with many mixed emotions and ethical conflicts. The latest story is from a January 3, 2003, article from ABC's news website on cloning that deals with five little piglets named Noel, Angel, Star, Joy, and Mary. Animals have a gene that humans (and monkeys) do not have. The gene causes animal organs to die quickly when transplanted into humans, therefore making animals unsuitable donors. These special cloned pigs were made missing a copy of that gene, essentially making them remarkably close matches for humans. The scientists wanted this done partly because pigs' organs are similar in size to humans, when looking at possible matches for transplantation.[11]

Animal-to-human transplants are called *xenotransplants*. There has often been controversy surrounding putting animal parts into people. Between people feeling squeamish about mixing species, and animal activists seeing these techniques as using animals as commodities and not living creatures, many people have reservations about the whole xenotransplant concept.

According to some scientists, now that a pig of this genetic engineering has been made, they wouldn't need to clone others, they would just inbreed those pigs. But that sparks an entirely new debate over genetic problems associated with inbreeding.

The fact that transplants are occurring frequently requires lawmakers to reevaluate decisions made in the past. One point to consider is ability to pay. Poor people who obey the law don't get free transplants. They must have insurance or some ability to pay or they will not get a transplant. You might wonder, "So why should taxpayers pay for incarcerated people? Wouldn't they rather just pay for a poor (yet law-abiding citizen) person who is in need?" The government should have to answer this valid question.

Organ donation is at a catastrophic low, with nearly 17 people dying each day while waiting for organs that never come. Should regular law-abiding citizens get passed up for someone who is not only incarcerated for violent crimes, but may be on death row or serving life sentences with no hope for parole? Are taxpayers expected to pay the astronomical fees for surgery and health maintenance posttransplant, then years later pay to have the person executed?

One Inmate's Story

There was a story on MSNBC's website titled "Convicted killer's transplant sparks ethical debate" about a woman named Carolyn Joy.[12] It started by revealing that Ms. Joy was a former prostitute convicted of murdering another prostitute in Omaha in 1983. She admitted her liver was ruined by an almost daily habit of heroin and alcohol abuse over a 9-year period.

Ms. Joy (at time of printing) was 49-years-old and had been drug free for almost 20 years. She knew that society would be offended that not only was she a convicted murderer, but that she was one who wanted a rare commodity, an organ transplant. She commented that she didn't know if she deserved a liver, but believed she'd paid her debt to society and now answered only to her family and God.

One thing that did unnerve her and keep her up at night was worrying about other people who needed livers. Currently, she is being evaluated to see if medically, she would be a good candidate. Carolyn Joy said she wanted a chance like everyone else, but if there were someone in more dire need than her next on the list, especially a young mother who had a real life and a child that depended on her, she'd gladly step aside.

Another hurdle she will have to overcome, even if it is decided that medically she should be added to the UNOS list, is that she must lose 30 pounds. Second, she'll have to get her diabetes under control before being considered for the transplant waiting list. She's already lost 70 pounds over the past 2 years, some because of illness. She's made a personal goal to overcome both challenges within 2 months. Ms. Joy was said to have made peace with the possibility she may not get the transplant and soon die and holds no one to blame.

People face prejudices every day, especially people with labels like "murderer." One man threatened to rip up his donor card if death-row inmates were allowed to get transplants. Although that person's strong statement may not be the norm, it raises a serious question. Is the general public open enough to ignore labels to see each potential recipient as merely a "patient"?

What really needs to be redefined is the 1976 ruling stating "The Right to Equal Medical Care." Yes, every American can be evaluated to see if they *could* be considered for a transplant. However, without ability to pay, they will *not* be put onto a transplant waiting list. Therefore, "Equal Medical Care" is a subjective phrase.

Half-million dollar elective surgeries seem a bit excessive to be considered "equal medical care." When the law was passed in the 1970s "equal medical care" meant routine checkups and everyday treatable conditions like high blood pressure, diabetes, and so forth. Transplants were not mainstream at the time like they are now. Once the cost of transplantation becomes closer to that of open-heart surgery, it might be fairly put in the "equal medical care" category. Until then, shouldn't it be considered "above and beyond" normal?

SHOULD AMERICAN CITIZENS GET TOP PRIORITY ON UNOS LIST?[13]

The Santillian's Story (February 2003)

Illegal immigrants in the United States getting organ transplants, like Jesica Santillan, the 17-year-old Mexican teen discussed in Chapter 9, has brought up this debate. Some transplant groups say it is only fair to give some organs to foreigners because they also donate organs to U.S. patients. UNOS allows for up to 5% of recipients to be from other countries. UNOS spokesman Joel Newman said, "Part of the rationale is that it may be hypocritical to accept donors who are not U.S. citizens, but not allow them to be transplant recipients."

A major factor in deciding who gets a transplant is the ability to pay. The federal government pays for some emergency medical services, but does not cover illegal immigrants who are unable to pay for a transplant. In the case of Jesica Santillan, she was covered under her mother's health insurance plan because her mom worked at Louisburg College, in Louisburg, North Carolina. The insurance would pay for 80% of the surgery, and a foundation created by family friend Mack Mahoney, would help the Santillans cover the rest of the costs incurred.

Not only did Jesica receiving a transplant cause a stir, but the fact that after a horrendous medical error (not matching blood types before surgery), which caused the donated organs to immediately reject, it took another 2 weeks to find matching organs. By then there really was no hope for Jesica, yet the medical community went ahead and performed another surgery, using two *more* lungs and *another* heart. In essence, between the botched first surgery and hopeless second surgery, the transplanted four lungs and two hearts may have saved at least six people.

To add to the situation, the newspapers wanted to get the story out immediately, so they didn't have time to wait for explanations regarding what really happened after Jesica died. All that was reported was that the family "refused to donate Jesica's organs." I was so outraged I couldn't even discuss it with people. I wanted to cry wondering what on Earth the family could have been thinking. I was angry with them for not giving back to the transplant community. Was their grief so immeasurable that they couldn't see past their anger? I couldn't see past their decision enough to investigate further, at least at first. When I cooled down enough, I decided to wait for the "real story" to come out. It was then that I sympathized with the family and its horrible situation.

As it turns out, according to the Santillans' friend Mr. Mahoney, Jesica's mother had asked doctors about donating the

Link to World Wide Transplant Centers
You can get to links for transplant centers in various countries all over the world. By going to the following link in 2004, I found two centers in Asia, 10 centers in Europe, two centers in Oceania, and 35 centers in North America. The link is: www.transweb.org/reference_sites/ centers.htm.

new heart and lungs as well as other organs. She was told the heart and lungs could not be reused and the kidneys and liver were ruined from being on life support too long. Other organs and tissues were so saturated with medications and antirejection drugs that they were not reusable, either. In addition, the family wanted an autopsy performed to learn the official "cause of death" of their daughter.

They received seething e-mails from all over the place once the first story appeared in the news, offering no explanation as to why the family did not donate Jesica's organs. Here were family members just needing to grieve, and they had to deal with paparazzi following them, making accusations about them, too. It was unfortunate on so many levels.

MOVIES, BOOKS, AND TV SHOWS THAT HAVE TRANSPLANT STORYLINES

Movies

I love movies. Who doesn't? They can make you laugh, cry, get mad, be scared, basically worry about someone else's life for a while and forget your own. When thinking back on some really good movies I've seen, some have had pretty serious subject matter. Read on about four movies whose storylines dealt with organ transplants. (These films are available at libraries or video stores.)

Steel Magnolias

Steel Magnolias, an oldie but a goodie, was Julia Roberts's first major role in a big-budget film with several Hollywood hitters. If you haven't seen it, you should. Julia plays a Southern belle with a mind of her own. She has diabetes and has been advised not to have children. Of course, she ignores doctors because babies are her number-one love. The pregnancy is successful, but is too hard on her kidneys, forcing her to begin dialysis. The dialysis becomes overwhelming and too time consuming, especially when trying to chase around her toddler. She decides to get a transplant. Because the waiting list is usually 3 to 5 years for a kidney, she is relieved and grateful to learn that her mother is a match who wants more than anything to be her daughter's donor.

The movie is about relationships of women, but the underlying story of transplantation is very moving. It shows how the women try to make light of the ominous situation, but her dad in the movie—played by Tom Skeritt—is so tense and angry, he doesn't like them teasing about it at all. In one scene, Julia's character and her brothers talk about what movie to watch, and one brother says, "How about 'A Tale of Two Kidneys,' um, I mean 'A Tale of Two Cities'." Julia bursts out laughing with that huge laugh of hers, and the dad has a fit.

John Q

John Q stars Denzel Washington, Anne Heche, James Woods, and Thandie Newton. It is about a family whose little boy collapses at his Little League baseball game. It turns out he will need a heart transplant. Because of miscommunications, it is discovered that the family's insurance policy will not cover the surgery and after exhausting all avenues, the dad (Denzel) snaps and locks down the emergency room at the hospital until the officials will give the boy a transplant.

It is a gut-wrenching movie that explores the problems with our health-care system and insurance companies in particular. It is action packed and emotional!

Return to Me

Return to Me stars Minnie Driver and David Duchovny. It is really a very funny movie, even though it is based on the premise of heart transplants. The secondary characters are what really make the film great. Carol O'Connor ("Archie Bunker" from the old television show *All in the Family*) is Driver's Irish grandpa who has raised her. He and his buddies are so funny and goofy that you'll want to watch them over and over again.

David Allen Grier plays Duchovny's best friend and a real "ladies man." Then there is Bonnie Hunt, from the TV series *Life with Bonnie* who plays Minnie's sister. She is sarcastic, yet loving. Bonnie Hunt actually wrote and directed the film, too! Jim Belushi plays Bonnie's husband and is his usual character, "a lovable, goofy, rough-around-the-edges guy." The cast cannot be beat, and the story is heart-warming (pun intended) and thought provoking, and, best of all, funny!

Blood Work

Blood Work stars Clint Eastwood, Angelica Houston, and Wanda De Jesus. Clint plays his usual, crusty, tough-guy, cop/FBI guy who has retired. This time, he has had a heart transplant, and finds out his donor was murdered. The donor's sister pleads with him to find the murderer. The story winds back to Clint in an interesting way. The reviews it got were positive for the actors, but the storyline was said to be predictable.

If you're looking for a show to feel a connection with, like one where you'll say, "Yes, that's exactly how I feel, too!" then my first choice would be for you to see *Return to Me*.

CELEBRITY PROFILES IN THE TRANSPLANT GAMES

Chris Klug is a professional snowboarder. In July 2000, he received a liver transplant after battling liver disease for 7 years. Only 5 months after his surgery, he was back on the snowboarding competition circuit, winning a World Cup victory in the parallel giant slalom.

At the 2002 Winter Olympics, he won the bronze medal in the men's parallel giant slalom. Chris says he thanks God every day for the second chance at life given to him by his donor family. He wants to help spread the life-saving message of organ donation and does this in part by taking part in the Transplant Games, which are held every 2 years. At the 2002 games, he participated in the Opening Ceremonies and the Donor Recognition Ceremony.[14]

Larry Hagman is an actor most known for television roles as J. R. Ewing on *Dallas* and Major Nelson on *I Dream of Jeannie*. He also appeared in movies including *Nixon* and *Primary Colors*, and authored his own autobiography titled *Hello Darlin'* about his professional and personal life.

Mr. Hagman had a liver transplant in 1995 and has been active in the transplant community ever since. He has been serving as honorary chairman of the National Kidney Foundation's U.S. Transplant Games since 1996.

According to Mr. Hagman, "the U.S. Transplant Games are a celebration of a second chance at life for transplant recipients from across the country."

Fernando Bryant is a star cornerback for the NFL's Jacksonville Jaguars. His brother Larry is alive today, thanks to a kidney transplant in 2001. Larry had battled kidney disease for 4 years before receiving this life-saving operation. Brother Fernando says, "[he] hopes to help draw attention to the urgent need for organ donors in this country."[15]

Books

Comparing Two Books: Raising the Dead *versus* Ethic of Organ Transplants: The Current Debate

There are two books that you should look into if you are really concerned about ethics of organ transplants. One is called *Raising the Dead: Organ Transplants, Ethics and Society*, by Ronald Munson, published by Oxford University

Press in 2002. The other book is called *The Ethics of Organ Transplants: The Current Debate*, edited by Arthur L. Caplan and Daniel H. Coehlo, published by Prometheus Books in 1998.[16] These two books really hash out tough questions like, "is a doctor's or lawyer's life more valuable than a bus boy's?" Because the professionals have money and insurance, they will be able to get a transplant if needed. The bus boy wouldn't be able to even consider such a costly option.

How about asking questions like whether inmates "deserve" a transplant, or if alcoholics "deserve" a new liver when theirs was ruined by self-infliction. The biggest concerns over ethics seem to really stem from how the organs are allocated, or passed out.

In Munson's book, *Raising the Dead*, he explains that a medical miracle does not happen with transplants, it is just trading one acute illness for a different chronic condition. Medical miracles are where a person's illness disappears. He agrees transplants work for now, but something more permanent and effective will hopefully be developed. Of course, that will probably come from a person's own DNA, requiring the use of embryonic stem cells and cloning technology, which will bring a whole slew of new issues to debate.

Munson's book tends to deal with a smaller number of topics, in terms of all the various avenues discussed regarding transplantation. However, it deals with the emotional side of the equation. It is aimed at people who don't have much experience with medical terms or ethical philosophies. It deals with people going through the transplant experience, which is similar to this book, designed for any type of reader, not just medical professionals.

Caplan and Coelho's book is aimed at medical professionals, although it contains a wealth of information for any type of reader, too. The difference is they cover a wide variety of and more in-depth information. They reprint articles from medical journals, so the overall writing and tone is different from a book for the "regular Joe or Jane" so to speak. That's not to say you need a medical degree to understand it, you will just have to read it more carefully than the other book.

A TRANSPLANT SURGEON BECOMES A U.S. SENATOR

U.S. Senator William Frist has been chosen as one of two alumni recipients of the 2003 Woodrow Wilson School of Public and International Affairs top honors.

Frist earned his medical degree from Harvard and went on to become a heart and lung transplant surgeon. Then, after joining the teaching faculty at Vanderbilt University Medical Center, the center became internationally renowned for multi-organ transplantation, under his leadership.

Frist was elected to the U.S. Senate in 1994, becoming the first practicing physician elected to the governing body since 1928! In the year 2000, he was elected to a second term by the largest margin ever received by a candidate for statewide election in the history of Tennessee.[17]

Television

ER

ER seems to have many storylines dealing with organ transplants each year. The problem is they usually make it so fast-paced that it really does not accurately portray the situation at hand when the question of donation comes about.

In one episode, a family was in a horrible car accident. The dad lived, the mom died, one boy needed a heart and lung transplant to survive, and the other brother was declared brain dead. The doctors battle back and forth with each other stating that one brother will have to save the other and that it is the only hope! They fight over getting the father to agree to the transplant and that's where the controversy lies.

In real life, there are proper steps that need to be taken. For example, while a family is allowed to request "directed donation" allowing an organ donation to go specifically from one family member to another family member, the organ procurement organization (OPO) would still need to be called first to make arrangements. Normally, after the OPO is contacted, and after consent has been given to donate, the United Network for Organ Sharing (UNOS) would be contacted. Later, a transplant team would need to be assigned and contacted.[18]

On *ER*, it wasn't specifically said that Dr. Elizabeth Corday would do the surgery, but as a viewer, I felt it was implied a little bit. At least, that is what I was led to believe. An emergency room doctor would not be able to perform transplant surgery!

But in usual *ER* fashion, Dr. Corday stands her ground and runs for the elevator to rush up to surgery. The father gives his consent, begging her to promise it will turn out all right, as the doors close with her grimacing and saying she can only do her best, she can't promise anything.

Whew, talk about gut wrenching! Although it makes for good TV, it's really not a very accurate description of the scenario because it ignores proper channels and protocol.

The biggest problem with such shows is that they are the place where many, many Americans get their knowledge and news. Viewers assume they are watching realistic situations. Viewers take the show at face value—as fact. After all, the show has medical advisors, so surely they would correct any mistakes, right? Wrong! The bottom line is that it is a *drama*. The point is to remember the show is *fiction*. Even if storylines are based on true concepts, the entire episode is not true.

Scrubs

Scrubs is an NBC comedy about medical residents. It does have emotional depth to it at times, too. In one episode, a person waiting for an organ donor made a valid yet simple point. She said that she was just tired of not knowing, she had even come to terms with death, but the uncertainty and waiting was the hardest part. She continued to wait on the list.

Ed

In one episode of *Ed*, another NBC show, an employer accused an employee of embezzling thousands of dollars. When the woman admitted she had embezzled money, they were stunned to learn she did it to help a dying man get a liver transplant.

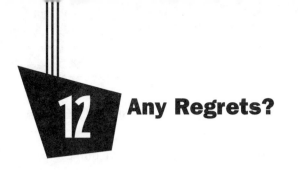

12 Any Regrets?

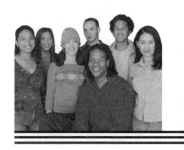

QUALITY OF LIFE VERSUS QUANTITY OF LIFE

First Ever Hand Transplant Recipient Wants It Taken Off

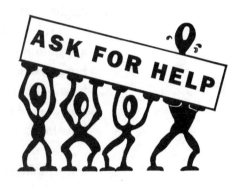

In a controversial experiment, the world's first hand transplant was performed in 1999 with not-so-wonderful results. In fact, the doctors and patient did not agree on the outcome. The *Hastings Center Report* discussed the problem of how surgeons and recipients might not be able to agree on the vague term "successful." For example, when discussing quality of life, a surgeon might feel a patient's quality of life has improved because of the mobility of a limb now available; whereas a patient might feel it's more of a hassle than it is worth. The antirejection drugs might make a patient sick or give unwanted side effects. Who has the right to say whether a recipient can give up and have an artificial limb amputated? Can a patient who volunteered to have a transplant decide when it has become too much for him or her?

When Clint Hallam agreed to be the first-ever hand transplant recipient, he knew it might be a rough ride. In reality, he had no idea. If the point of transplantation is "quality of life," and Clint felt he didn't have it, couldn't he decide to have the donor tissues removed?

After surgery, he had symptoms from pins and needles to a kind of burning sensation. Doctors told Clint it was from going off his immunosuppressant drugs. But Clint said the drugs were causing chronic diarrhea and frequent bouts of flu. His quality of life was not good because of it.

The surgeons were angry, stating that they gave him the chance of a lifetime and he ruined it and he was a bad example. They commented on their strict selection process, and how they were disappointed that they somehow chose the wrong patient.

Wow, talk about harsh! Those doctors were mad. Time, money, experimentation, trials, and tribulations went into making the hand transplant happen. But when all is said and done, if the surgeons were the ones with constant flu symptoms, chronic diarrhea, and pain and burning in their body, they might react differently.

It is hard to say what you might do unless you are actually in a situation yourself. It's easy to say, "Oh, I'd just stick it out and hope it all got better," or "Hey, he agreed to the experiment, so he should just do what the doctors want." In reality, you just don't know what you could or could not withstand and for how long.

Yes, the idea and surgery were a *huge* gamble that unfortunately did not pay off. The surgeons and physicians needed to take a step back and decide where to go next. The world's best breakthroughs and discoveries usually come from initial failures. It was the first go-around with transplanting a hand. Surely the experience garnished tons of valuable information, so not all was lost! In February 2001, surgeons removed Mr. Hallam's transplanted hand.[1]

SUCCESS? YOU BE THE JUDGE

Since that first experiment involving a hand transplant went awry, there have been two successful hand transplants, but controversy still ensues. Some doctors feel this procedure is still premature, and that having to take strong immunosuppressant drugs, which can have potentially fatal side effects, is not a risk to take because hands are not necessary for survival.

Yes, hands do add to quality of life tremendously; however, until more research can be done to improve the antirejection medications, some doctors say hand transplantation should still be considered experimental.

CYSTIC FIBROSIS COMPLICATION TAKE WOMAN'S LIFE AFTER SUCCESSFUL TRANSPLANT

Kimberly Miles was a 33-year-old a woman whose mom and friend both donated parts of their lungs to her because it was her only hope of survival. (Kimberly's sister Tammy and a friend DorMae Gebhardt, both in their early 30s with families of their own, offered to be donors as well.)

Doctors didn't feel Kimberly would live long enough to receive a cadaveric donor, which is why she needed lungs donated from live donors. She had cystic fibrosis (CF), a disorder that causes patients to have mucus build up in their lungs. The constant clearing of mucus scars the lungs and eventually wears them out, causing a person to essentially suffocate.

Cystic fibrosis complications can also cause a failing digestive system, which is what happened to Kimberly. Just two years after her transplant, which was technically a success since the lungs were functioning, digestive complications killed her.

The entire last two years of her life were filled with various health problems, so although the procedure added two whole years to her life, they wouldn't be considered "quality years." Both donors said they didn't regret going through the operation. It was Kimberly's only chance of survival, so they took it. The only thing they regret was her not getting quality of life out of it.[2]

The doctors agreed and said, in hindsight, because her quality of life really wasn't improved they would *not* do it over again. The problem with CF is doctors *don't* know who will have complications of the disease and who will not. Some patients like Jim Leman, profiled in Chapter 2, have no problems, even though he also had been living with cystic fibrosis for many years.

Quality Versus Quantity
One of the biggest debates over organ transplantation is that its sole purpose is to increase *quality* of life, not just quantity! As you can see in this chapter, not everyone who has had a transplant would do it over again.

185

WHY I SAID, "NO THANKS. I'LL PASS"—DAD WHO REFUSES TO BE PUT ON UNOS LIST

Alpha-1 Antitrypsin Deficiency

Michelle and Ed Eymer are the founders and managers of the Alpha Wings BMX Racing Team. Ed was diagnosed with Alpha-1 Antitrypsin deficiency (known as "Alpha-1" or "AAT deficiency") several years ago. He was also diagnosed with emphysema, asthma, and bronchitis. Now in his 40s, he has been on oxygen for 7 years. Due to the lack of knowledge of Alpha-1, it took four different doctors over a period of 2 years to diagnose Ed. By this time, he had already lost 80% of his lung function. Alpha-1 can be detected by a simple blood test.

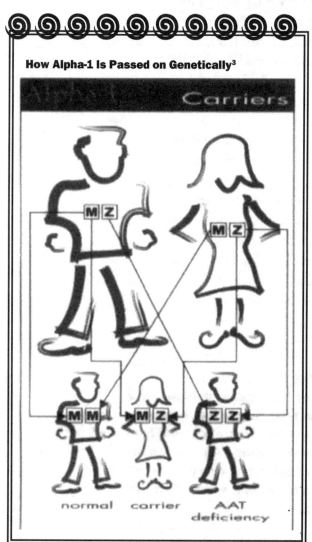

How Alpha-1 Is Passed on Genetically[3]

normal   carrier   AAT deficiency

Three of the Alpha Wings' team members (Jayson, Mathew, and Jonathan Eymer) are called "MZ carriers" of Alpha-1. As carriers, they will need to be concerned as to how this deficiency will affect them in later years and also whether they will pass Alpha-1 on to their children.

Studies suggest that 80,000 to 100,000 Americans (and similar numbers in Europe) have severe AAT deficiency, which would equal approximately 1 in every 3,000 people. However, approximately 95% of those people who are estimated to have AAT deficiency have not even been diagnosed! An estimated 25 million people in the United States are undetected carriers. Most often patients are misdiagnosed with asthma or smoking-related chronic obstructive pulmonary disease (COPD). You can visit www.alphaone.org to learn more.[4]

The Eymer brothers, who really loved BMX racing, formed the Alpha Wings team in the spring of 2001. (*BMX* stands for *bicycle motocross*, which is an extreme sport where riders race around a dirt track made up of huge hills, jumps, and berms. Riders range from 3 years old to almost 60 years old, and include people who can ride a two-wheeler and want to race. There are outdoor and indoor tracks so riders can race all year long.)

The two national BMX leagues have tracks all over the country. To find out more about racing, check out the National Bicycle League at www.nbl.org and the American Bicycle Association at www.ababmx.com.

The kids wanted to name their team Alpha Wings to help promote awareness of Alpha-1, in honor of their friends and family who have been stricken with the genetic disease. They even visit schools to promote awareness of the disease. They show their equipment, jerseys, and trophies, too!

Alpha Wings BMX Racing Team

The Alpha Wings team is made up of 23 riders in various classes, or skill levels, and ages, ranging from 6-year-old riders to 43-year-old riders, both male and female. In the 2001–2002 season, the team placed fourth (of 24 teams locally) in the top-10 highest scoring teams for the American Bicycle League (ABA) at its local track. In the National Bicycle League (NBL), they had riders place first in the fall series and fifth, seventh, and ninth for the state of Illinois competition. State races are really big deals, where hundreds of racers of all ages gather for the big yearly competition. In the 2002–2003 winter season, they were number one at the Elkhorn, Wisconsin, track with 15 teams competing.

Ed and Michelle Eymer are team managers who promote good sportsmanship, good attitude, team spirit, hard work, and honesty. "We are very proud of all the Alpha Wings riders for their hard work on and off the track in spreading their wings to help promote the awareness of this disease," said manager Michelle Eymer. "Special thanks go out to those who believed in us and helped us get our team off the ground."

If you are interested in helping the Alpha Wings continue to spread the awareness, please contact: Alpha Wings, c/o Ed and Michelle Eymer, 14630 Wadsworth Road, Wadsworth, IL 60083. E-mail: eymersalpha5@aol.com or visit their website and www.alphawingsbmx.com.

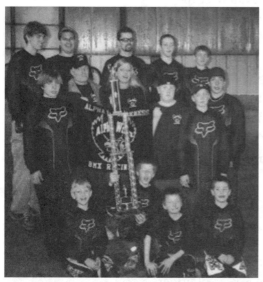

Ed and Michelle Eymer with the Alpha Wings BMX team

Ed Eymer has chosen *not* to be a lung transplant candidate. There are many things he does and enjoys in life and he has decided, after discussing it with his family, that a transplant is just not the right option for him for now.

Seven years ago, Ed was given a 2-year prognosis of survival without a lung transplant. He has not had one and is still alive today. That's not to say his life has not been affected. Although he met the requirement of total disability by the time he was diagnosed with Alpha-1, Ed continued to work for 5 more years, until 2001. Work eventually become too difficult, so he had to retire.

Michelle, his wife, had recently retired from her job (at only 43 years old) to be with him and help when he was ill. She plans on working a home profession so she can be close to Ed.

One complication Ed has experienced is that his heart is three times larger because of stress put on it from his lungs. If he receives new lungs that are healthy, the heart should return to normal size. Even a common cold can be a dangerous illness for Ed; because his liver doesn't make enzymes, his lungs cannot fight off germs that a cold brings. A cold virus in the lungs causes lung tissue damage.

The most common signs and symptoms of Alpha-1 are:[5]

- Family history of lung disease or liver disease
- Shortness of breath or awareness of one's breathing
- Decreased exercise tolerance
- Nonresponsive asthma or year-round allergies
- Recurring respiratory infections
- Rapid deterioration of lung function without a history of significant smoking
- Chronic liver problems
- Elevated liver enzymes

Please share this information with your friends. Early detection may add years to an Alpha-1's life!

New Treatments, No Cure Yet

Although there is no cure for Alpha-1, a treatment (which is expensive) has been successful for Ed so far. Once a week, he has to have an IV (intravenous) dose of Prolastin (human plasma) that slows down the deterioration of the lungs, caused by Alpha-1.

Once Ed had a bad reaction to a medication called Prednisone. It gave him osteoporosis (brittle bones). He had one incident where his chest muscles tightened so much and squeezed his lungs that he couldn't move or get air. The paramedics tried giving him oxygen, but his body didn't react. Next they gave him a steroid shot to relax the muscles, which had gone into spasms, causing hundreds of stress fractures in his ribs. Bone scans showed high risk of fracturing his lumbar, or lower back, so he was unable to use an instrument called "the vest." The vest is worn by some patients to pump the chest to break up the mucous and clear out the lungs. This helps to avoid pneumonia. Ed was then given calcium, which other people with Alpha-1 usually respond to, but it did not help.

In January 2003, Ed started a new FDA-approved drug called *Forteo*, which promotes bone growth. The goal is to take it for 19–24 months, then patients are supposedly finished and won't need it again. The only side effect Ed has experienced on this drug so far is stomach problems.

Michelle said she and Ed have discussed if there ever would be a time for a transplant. She said, "Yes, if he got sick enough where that was his only chance of survival, and he was simply incapacitated without it, he would want to be put on the UNOS list. But for now, he is maintaining his health adequately (he feels) and will just leave things as they are for now."

As of 2004, Ed and Michelle's boys were 10, 12, and 16 years old. I asked Michelle if the risks of Ed *not* having a transplant concerned her, being a parent with three kids. She said she talks to him openly and honestly and will stand by him and respect whatever decisions he makes. If the time comes when he feels he needs a transplant, she will support that decision, too.

It is a very difficult decision whether or not to be put on a recipient waiting list. It's not always a simple "cut and dried" decision. Ed's story shows you that you just never know what to think. He was given a 2-year life expectancy and has happily outlived that prognosis given by doctors. However, Ed is one of the lucky ones.

"Even though the financial stress is a great burden on a disabled person," Michelle said, "as a family we feel that the quality of life is what is important. Plus, the importance of spreading the awareness of Alpha-1 can help add years to an Alpha's life."

After reading about the stresses and potential hazards, not to mention financial and emotional strain, it demonstrates that transplantation is not the right decision for everyone. It should be discussed and decided on a case-by-case basis.

A MOTHER'S LOVE, A YOUNG MAN'S DECISION, AND A BOOK

Tim's Place is a book by Judy Fringuello about her son Tim's battle against kidney disease. When he was 13 years old, he had one of the early kidney transplants and his mother Judy was the donor. The transplant took place in 1970.[6]

Seven years later, his kidney started rejecting and his siblings got tested to see if any of them were matches for him. One of his sisters was a match, but Tim didn't want to go through a transplant again and decided to go on dialysis instead. Knowing this decision would surely shorten his life, his mom objected, but he was a 20-year-old young adult by then and had to make the decision for himself.

As the years went on, in his 20s and 30s he continued to do things he loved, like riding motorcycles with his friends. But Tim had lost a lot of strength and energy, so he couldn't work a regular job anymore. He lived with his parents and did work around the house for them, like carpentry projects. He replaced their garage with a shed he built himself, adding a sign that said, "Tim's Place."

The hardest times for him were watching friends get married and have kids. He knew that he probably wouldn't experience those things for himself. But when his best friend had a little boy, he named him Tim.

His mother Judy kept journals for each of her children as they grew up. When Tim was 38 years old, he died and Judy decided to honor his memory. Tim made his own decision and lived out his life as he wanted to.

Judy wanted to try to help other parents get through their experiences of having children with chronic illnesses. She decided to write a book about Tim based on events from her journal. Judy's goal was to give others hope and help them keep faith. The cover of her book has an illustration of that shed Tim built, which is still intact today behind her home as a tribute to him. The sign still reads "Tim's Place."

You can order a copy of the book *Tim's Place* online at www. NuLeafPublishing.com.

Judy mentions the importance of having a support system. She recommends having someone at home, or at least someone going through a similar situation, who can empathize with you. As you've heard over and over from professionals, recipients, and other family members, you simply cannot go through this type of experience alone.

You need to trust your own instincts, especially when medical recommendations are concerned. Nobody knows your parent (or yourself if you're the recipient) better than you, so if you don't agree with a doctor's recommendations, tell that doctor. You have every right to question medical advice or even get a second or third or however many opinions you feel necessary.

One Daughter's Feelings
"I was very upset, my dad did not let me know (the transplant was going on) until my mom was in surgery. I was in Florida and my mom was in Illinois. When my dad said to me (on the phone) 'sit down,' I knew something was wrong. I began shaking and crying. I was a mess. I just did not know what to think," said Ann, a 22-year-old whose mother had a double-lung transplant. "My brother flew home that night and was there for the wait, but my dad did not want me to miss (my college) classes. I ended up missing them anyways. I stuck by my friends the whole time."

Ann also said, "I was upset that I wasn't allowed to be there during the operation and I let my father know, but he disagreed with me, so that was the end of it. It would have meant a lot more to me if I flew home that night."

HELPING POTENTIAL DONORS SPEAK
THEIR FINAL WISHES

While waiting for a kidney transplant, Janelle London said, "I wanted to turn it into something positive by getting involved . . . and help other patients." She volunteers with various kidney transplant and organ donation organizations during her free time. By educating the public about the organ shortage, she feels she is helping others as well as herself. She has several different projects in the works.

One of the more gutsy and innovative ideas is a toll-free number that callers can record their wishes to be an organ donor, and say any other last words to their families, in case they should die in an accident. The family can access the recording and listen to the deceased person's final wishes so they know firsthand what their loved one would have wanted.[7]

Janelle has many unique projects going on any given moment. She also swam the San Francisco Bay on October 4, 1997, and August 2, 1998. She believed swimming from Alcatraz to San Francisco, while undergoing dialysis treatments, could show other dialysis patients that determination can lead to healthy and active lifestyles. Janelle is an attorney in San Francisco, California, and received a kidney transplant on April 21, 1999. She is profiled on the www.UNOS.org website.

Ever hear that expression, "You can lead a horse to water, but you can't make it drink"? It means that no matter how badly you want people to do something, even if it is for their own good, *they* have to want to do it themselves or it won't get done.

My friend "Tammy's" mother was like that. Tammy didn't want to speak in this book specifically because her experience is still too painful to discuss, but said I could give the gist of the situation. Her mom needed a kidney transplant and was on the UNOS waiting list. She would not allow any of her children to be tested for compatibility. As a result, she passed away in 1999 while still waiting.

Although her children are still mourning the loss, I had to wonder if their mom gave a reason for not letting them get tested. Tammy said that because she wasn't married, and her mother knew she wanted kids someday, her mom didn't want to risk taking away that option by leaving her with one kidney. Because her other siblings were already married and had children, she didn't want to risk their lives or health since they have young kids to raise.

As an outsider, I think that is a very selfless and honorable decision. But as a person who still has both parents, my heart aches for the family. One argument is that, being adults, her kids should have been able to decide if they wanted to donate or not. But being their mother, and the potential recipient, it was ultimately the mother's decision to accept or not accept such a gift.

There are always risks for surgeries and the mother would have been devastated if anything happened to her children a result of a transplant, so you can see now why she might have made the decision she did.

MEDICAL MISTAKES: HUMAN ERRORS

A 17-year-old girl was given a 6-month life expectancy without a heart-lung transplant. Her prospects were not good, because she had type O blood.[8]

As mentioned before, type O blood can be universally donated, meaning it can be put in any other blood type's body. However, type O blood can only receive other type O blood. It cannot substitute any other type. The patient with type O blood has less opportunity to find a matching donor.

A miracle seemed to happen when an organ bank called with a heart and lung match. The girl was contacted and prepped for surgery immediately. The surgery took place quickly, and as it was ending, doctors discovered the donor organs, while properly labeled as type A, did NOT match the girl's blood type, which was type O. By the time the error was discovered, her body was already rejecting the new heart and lungs.

She was immediately listed for a second transplant operation, which she received 2 weeks later. But by then, it was too late to save her. The medical team told her family about the human error immediately, and that the first operation failed solely because of unmatched blood types.

Regrets and Hope

There is a twofold question regarding regret. First, does the family regret the daughter's surgery? And second, many critics question, should Americans have priority for transplants, since this patient had not been a U.S. citizen?

Transplant groups point out that it's only fair to give some organs to foreigners because they also donate organs to U.S. patients. (However, it's worth noting that the girl wasn't merely foreign, she was here illegally. She didn't go through proper channels like other "foreigners" go through when coming to America.)

Last, the second transplant brings up one more issue on regrets. After such a lengthy amount of time on anti-rejection drugs that obviously were not working, should a whole set of three life-saving organs (one heart and two lungs that could have saved three or more lives) been given to a patient with virtually no statistical chance of survival? Was it done as a gesture to show the family the medical professionals' regrets over their error? Then did doctors simply go above and beyond what was medically possible to try to right the wrong that had occurred?

Whether we can accept it or not, people make mistakes. It's horrible to have to face that fact when the medical profession is concerned. However, the facts are the facts, humans still perform medicine, *not* machines. In a report issued in 1999, the Institute of Medicine estimated that between 44,000 and 98,000 people die each year from medical errors.

Priorities need to be reassessed in many fields in America. Health and education are two areas that need some serious revamping. These two areas specifically concern you, readers of this book. And knowledge is power! If you want things to change, then you help change them. You have a voice and a mind, and can think up great ideas, so use them and make yourself heard.

GET INSPIRED

"How can I make a difference, I'm just a teenager?" you may think. Do you need inspiration? Be sure to review the next chapter of this book very carefully. It's called "How *You* Can Make a Difference," and you can make all the difference in the world! Who knows what amazing thing you might accomplish in your life? You might be the next great inventor or discover something to save the world. Anything is possible. But nothing will change if you don't try.

13 How *You* Can Make a Difference

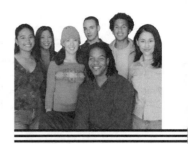

GET A DONOR CARD

Although you might not be going across the country to spread awareness of organ and tissue donation, there are a variety of ways in which you can help to circulate the information. Read on and get inspired on how to do just that.

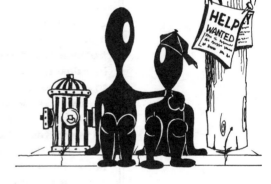

Personally, you can help by signing the back of your driver's license if you're old enough to have one. Then, you should get a separate donor card as well. It is very important to share your decision/wishes with family members. It's as easy as copying a page from this book, filling it out, and carrying it with you.

Fold Here

UNIFORM DONOR CARD   Carry with your driver's license

Name:_____

In the hope that I may help others, I hereby make this anatomical gift, if medically acceptable, to take effect upon my death. The words and marks below indicate my desire:

I Give: (a) _____ any needed organ or tissues
             (b) _____ only the following organs or tissues:

_____
specify organ(s) or tissue(s):

for the purpose of transplantation, therapy, medical research or education.

Limitations or special wishes, if any:_____
_____

Signed by the donor and the following witnesses in the presence of each other:

_____
Signature of the Donor   Date of Birth

_____
City/State   Date Signed

Witness: _____

Witness: _____

This is a legal document under the uniform Anatomical Gift Act or similar laws.

Note: If you are under 19 years of age, please have your signature witnessed by a parent or guardian.

TO NEXT-OF-KIN: Please notify physician that I am a donor.

PLATFORM—ORGAN DONATION AWARENESS

Tina Marie Sauerhammer, a Korean American, who had been Miss Madison, was crowned Miss Wisconsin in 2003 and went on to become the third runner up in the 2004 Miss America Pageant. She was the youngest person to graduate from UW–Madison Medical School at only 22 years old. No doctor has ever entered the Miss Wisconsin pageant, let alone won it!

Miss Wisconsin's father, Randy, died in 2001 from Wagner's disease, a rare disease that attacks every main organ. He died on his 45th birthday while waiting for a kidney transplant.

Because of his rare blood type and poor health, they didn't expect to get a call from the transplant center until he was moved up the list more. One night, after a preliminary pageant competition in June 2001, the family returned home to an urgent message on their answering machine, saying a donor had been found. Randy was not wearing his pager. By the time he called the center, it was too late, the kidney had been given to someone else before it expired.

Randy Sauerhammer was a huge influence in Tina Marie's life, helping her with medical school and even helping her with all the contests she had entered over the years. That is why Tina decided to go forth with pageantry, to give back to her father. Her platform was to bring attention to the urgent need of organ and tissue donation.[1]

BE SURE YOUR WISHES ARE KNOWN: TELL YOUR FAMILY

What would happen if you were critically injured and declared brain dead? The hospital wouldn't just check your wallet and say, "Oh, she signed her license. Now we don't have to ask her parents if they'd consider donating their daughter's organs or tissues. It says 'yes' right here." Although seven states currently accept a signed driver's license as a legal and binding decision on being an organ donor, the other 43 states have different policies.

In the United States, 42 of the 50 states, plus the District of Columbia have a place on the driver's license where it indicates your wish to be an organ donor. The only eight states that don't have it yet are: Alaska, California, Kansas, Kentucky,

Michigan, Nebraska, New York, and Oklahoma. If you live in one of these states, try writing letters to such government officials as your secretary of state or your governor. Do you know their names? You can find that information easily by going to your state's website. Not sure of the link? Just go to www.google.com to search for the information.

Do a presentation about signing the back of your license for all the driver's ed. classes in your school.

LEGALLY, DO *YOU* HAVE THE FINAL SAY IN WHAT HAPPENS WHEN YOU DIE?

No. If you are in a brain-dead state, the next of kin has to sign a waiver for you to be an organ or tissue donor. Your wishes are not necessarily going to be carried out unless a parent (or next of kin) signs the permission forms granting the hospital the right to take your organs for donation. Of the 80% of people who sign up to be organ donors, only a small percentage of those actually donate. Only approximately 20% are used as donors because family members are so unsure as to what the potential donor wanted. The subject was never discussed, or the person's wishes were not made clear. Many people just say they don't know, so they don't want to give permission for donation.

That's why it is so important for you to not only share your wishes with your parents and other family members, but to reinforce those wishes to them, so it sticks in their mind. When life-and-death situations occur and parents get the call they all dread, "There's been a horrible accident, and you need to come to the hospital" the last thing they will be able to comprehend is "brain dead" and "possible organ donor." If this is something that has been discussed several times, then it will be an automatic response versus an outrageous and impossible request to even consider. If you truly wish to allow yourself to be a donor, should the horrible circumstance arise, make your wishes clear to your family.

199

KIDS KARE

The website www.kidscare.org is made by kids and is for kids. Plus, there are tons of great things to click on. Three of the best links I recommend from the Kids Kare site are:

1. Recipes—"The hottest rock group around, 'Spice Rack,' is here to teach you some radical recipes and tell you some foods you should eat before and after organ transplants!" Then you click where it says to.

2. Net Pals—"Hey kids! Do you want an Internet pen pal? If you do then you have come to the right place! To receive a Net Pal all you have to be is a kid!" Then you click where it says to.

3. Scrapbook—This has pictures of the kids of various ages, even teens, working on the website and going to competitions for Community Problem Solving (CmPS).

SOME ORGANIZATIONS TO BE AWARE OF

Kids Kare

Kids Kare is an award-winning public education program for kids made up by kids (and some teens). The kids who started it are from Merritt Island, Florida. Their website features a continuing story with characters receiving transplants. The goal of the website is to make kids aware of what organ and tissue donation is and "to help kids understand that organ donation is the best kind of sharing in the world!"

The Kids Kare website is geared toward younger children more than toward teens, but is still worth checking out. Categories on the home page include scrapbook, recipes, net pals, e-mail, "kool links," special thanks, and how to join the club. You can check out the site at www.kidskare.org.

"KEEP" Organization

Another public education program is called KEEP, (Kidney Early Evaluation Program). It is a free health-screening program designed to identify and educate people who are at an increased risk for developing kidney disease. Some of those at increased risk include: persons with diabetes and/or high blood pressure or those who have a first-degree relative—parent, grandparent, or sibling—with high blood pressure, diabetes, or chronic kidney failure.

NATIONAL MINORITY DONOR AWARENESS DAY

You can spread awareness of National Minority Donor Awareness Day (NMDAD). It is observed each year on August 1 and is an intensive awareness campaign reaching out to minorities of all ethnic groups. NMDAD focuses on the various (organ/tissue donation) fears and obstacles directly related to minorities. The objective is to promote healthy living and disease prevention and to increase the number of people who sign donor cards, have family discussions, and actually become donors. In addition, NMDAD increases national awareness of the disproportionate rates of hypertension, diabetes, and kidney and other diseases that affect minorities at a much higher incidence than its counterparts. Also, this day of observance increases awareness of the behaviors that can lead to the need for transplantation, such as smoking, alcohol and substance abuse, and poor nutrition.

This particular day highlights donor families of all ethnic groups across the country including: African Americans, Hispanics/Latinos, Asians, Alaska Natives, Pacific Islanders, and Native Americans. Activities held in observance of NMDAD include: prayer breakfast, health walks, donor drives at shopping malls, and tree-planting ceremonies.[3]

According to a study by the Robert Wood Johnson University Hospital, 60% of African Americans said they would not donate their organs because they do *not* trust the medical system. Many people are uncomfortable signing an organ donor card because they fear doctors will not work as hard to save their own life. If donation is something you want to do, don't keep it a secret!

KEEP participants have their weight and blood pressure checked. Blood and urine are collected from individuals who require further testing after the initial weight and blood pressure check. An onsite doctor goes over the results with participants. Everyone will receive educational material about preventing and treating kidney disease, high blood pressure, and diabetes.[2]

Coalition on Donation

Coalition on Donation was founded by UNOS in 1992. Its purpose is to educate the public about organ and tissue donation, clear up misconceptions about donation, and to inspire everyone to feel comfortable making the choice to donate.

The Coalition on Donation is a nonprofit alliance of 49 national organizations and 49 local coalitions. The goal is to make sure everyone in the United States understands the need for organ and tissue donation and accepts donation as a fundamental human responsibility.

START A LOCAL SUPPORT GROUP FOR TEENS AND YOUNG ADULTS IN YOUR AREA

Who says you can't start your own organization? Just because you are young, it doesn't mean you are not able to start something up. Get some friends to help you. You could start a local support group easily by hanging up posters around school or church (after getting permission from the place you would like to hold meetings.) You could even go to local retailers (such as the grocery store, pizza parlor, dry cleaners, or other business establishments) to get out a simple message of dates and times your group will meet. Address it to kids your age who are going through some aspect of organ transplantation or a donor situation. You could even put up a sign at your local clinic or at the office your parent goes to for checkups.

Whether a parent was a donor, or a sibling placed on a waiting list to have a transplant, or even if you yourself are the

Now Is the Time
As a college student, you will have the time, confidence, and contacts to make a real difference in your community. Organ and tissue awareness is sadly quite absent on many college campuses in Illinois and around the country. There are many different ways you can help increase awareness about organ and tissue donation on your campus and in your community. To learn more about how you can increase donation from your campus, contact Gift of Hope (Illinois Coalition) at 1-888-307-DON8.

one who needs a transplant, reaching out to others in the community could be just what you *and* they need to help them through this experience.

Finding an Advisor

You might want to ask an adult you trust, like a school counselor or teacher or social worker, to be the group's advisor. Perhaps this person would be willing to be the meeting facilitator and help run the discussions. With emotional topics, groups can easily get off on tangents or even become very negative about what's wrong with the current transplant system. Granted, it should be an avenue for people to vent their frustrations and fears, but you don't want an angry mob scene, where everyone is just jumping in telling his or her own version of "you think you have it bad, listen to this!" That would be very counterproductive, especially because the biggest help to families going through organ transplant situations is to keep a positive attitude.

High Praise

"I think this book [*Organ Transplants: A Survival Guide for The Entire Family: The Ultimate Teen Guide*] should be given to patients by physicians; also, so that children, teens, and young adults can be educated about transplantation and to know it can and will be an emotional time for all," says Celeste, double-lung recipient and mother of a 19- and 23-year-old.

One of the biggest things you can do for yourself and others is help educate on transplantation. As the saying goes, "Knowledge *is* power!"

It seems cliché, but sayings like "mind over matter" or "think positive" can help lift your spirits and keep you and your family going on the quest for survival. If everyone always talks about the negatives, and the "one and a million shot" there is to match tissues and blood type, and be in good health, potential transplant recipients and their families would get discouraged and depressed. That could lead the patient's health to decline. Attitude and hopefulness are ultimately what will get you and your parents to survive and come out on top. Outlook really increases the chance of survival.

A DONOR FATHER WORKING TO MAKE A DIFFERENCE

Stephen Oelrich, the sheriff of Alachua County, Florida, has set up a campaign to help solve the problem of donor shortage. After the death of his 18-year-old son, Nick, in 1995, Sheriff Oelrich established the Gift of Life Foundation of the National Sheriffs' Association, NSA. You can see the website by going to www.nsagiftoflife.org.

Sheriff Oelrich's office holds an annual Nick Oelrich "Gift of Life" Golf Classic each fall. The tournament in 2001 raised more than $10,000 to support the projects of the Gift of Life Foundation.

For more information about the Gift of Life Foundation of the National Sheriffs' Association contact Linda White, Public Information Bureau Chief at (352) 955-1805.

NATIONAL SHERIFF'S ASSOCIATION—GIFT OF LIFE

The NSA Gift of Life organizes help from law enforcement communities throughout the country to promote organ and tissue donation. At NSA's annual convention in Columbus, Ohio, in June 2002, sheriffs encouraged their employees to consider the option of organ donation by distributing donor cards with employee paychecks. This is an excellent, yet simple, idea that you could share with employers. See if they would consider distributing donor cards in employees' paychecks at your work, too!

JOURNALING AND/OR ART

Try to keep a journal of your thoughts, feelings, and experiences throughout the entire process. You can write poetry, draw artwork, or even write in it like a diary. In time, you might be willing to share it with others who might feel like they're the only one with those thoughts and feelings. Once your parent or other loved one has survived surgery and a few years have passed, it might be helpful for you to revisit your journal. It will serve as a gentle reminder of just how far you and your family have come. It really does help keep things in perspective once your life gets back to its normal routine.

TRIO
The Transplant Recipients International Organization (TRIO), Inc. posted this on their website: "United Airlines Miles Urgently Needed! Donate your United Airlines Frequent Flyer miles so TRIO can keep providing FREE transplant-related air travel."[4]

START LOCAL AWARENESS CAMPAIGN

National Donate Life Month is observed every April. Plan ahead to make a big deal about it. You can design an ad for your local papers and ask them to donate space for a public service announcement regarding National Donate Life Month. You can design your own special posters for local businesses, or go to the UNOS website (www.unos.org) to see if there is a uniform logo or ad it prefers to be used. Dig around and do some research on the requirements and how you can personalize an ad for your community.

And the Winner Is . . .
Illinois has a contest for kids making posters to promote organ and tissue donation. In 2002, a 17 year old won, and in 2003 a 7 year old won. The posters are displayed at libraries and on the website www.cyberdriveillinois.com.

Maybe include a picture of some local organ recipients or donors, maybe even your parent! Have them highlighted as Neighbor of the Week in some local newspaper neighborhood section. Use your imagination! The sky is the limit.

A wonderful way to raise local awareness is to promote the website from the Gift of Life Donor Program. The website (www.donors1.org) has a special section on the Transplant Games, highlighted in Chapters 8 and 11. The website also has a section of donor tributes called "Donor Families: We Remember Them," which shares photos and profiles of donors young and old alike. It is a wonderful way to remember your loved ones and show the world what wonderful people they were. What a great way to honor their memory!

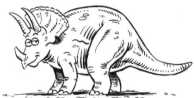

ONE DONORSAUR

CAN HELP MORE THAN 50 TRANSPLANT RECIPIENTS

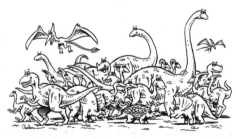

In 2003, Gift of Hope Organ and Tissue Donor Network worked with 309 families who said "yes" to organ donation. Through their generous decision to donate life, Gift of Hope provided 972 lifesaving organs for transplant.

In addition, 870 families consented to tissue donation, allowing tens of thousands of patients to receive medical transplants of bone, heart valves, and other tissues. You could help increase those already impressive numbers by getting involved in the regional organ bank in your area.

By volunteering your time or talents in whatever way the organizations see fit, great things can be accomplished. Search the web, or even your local yellow pages, to find an organ bank in your area.

Thank you for taking the time to learn about organ and tissue donation. I wish you and your family health and happiness for years to come.

Write Your State Rep.
There was a semipostal stamp for Organ and Tissue Donation you can see at www.trioweb.org. Write your state representative today to ask for reissue of the stamp!

FUN QUIZ FROM GIFT OF HOPE ORGAN AND TISSUE DONOR NETWORK[5]

Now that you've read a ton of information on organ donation and transplantation, and a bit on tissue donation, too, let's see what you remember! (You can find the answers in the back of the book.)

1. Only rich or famous people get organs.
   True   False

2. How old do you have to be to be a donor?
   16   Any age
   30   85

3. Circle the six organs that can be transplanted:
   Heart   Stomach
   Nose   Pancreas
   Lungs   Liver
   Kidneys   Mouth
   Brain   Small intestine

4. Gift of Hope Organ and Tissue Donor Network supplies organs for transplant and provides _____ for the community and health care professionals.
   Lunch   Money
   Education

5. It is illegal to sell organs:
   True   False

6. All major religions support organ and tissue donation:
   True   False

7. How many people are currently on the national transplant waiting list?
   10   4,100
   84,000   One Million

8. What is the best way to be sure that you will become a donor?
   Sign a donor card   Tell your family
   Hire a sky writer   Rent a billboard

FUN QUIZ ANSWERS

1. Only rich or famous people get organs.
   False. Organs are matched through a national computer-based system based on size, blood type, time on the waiting list, location, and many other factors. Money or celebrity status does not matter.
2. How old do you have to be to be a donor?
   Any age.
3. 6 organs that can be transplanted:
   Heart, lungs, kidneys, pancreas, liver, and small intestine.
4. Gift of Hope Organ and Tissue Donor Network supplies organs for transplant and provides *education* for the community and healthcare professionals.
5. It is illegal to sell organs.
   True. It is a federal law that organs cannot be sold—not even on E-Bay!
6. All major religions support organ and tissue donation.
   True. All major religions believe that organ and tissue donation is the ultimate act of love and kindness toward others.
7. How many people are currently on the national transplant waiting list?
   84,000. (There are 4,400 in Illinois.)
8. What is the best way to be sure that you will become a donor?
   Tell your family.

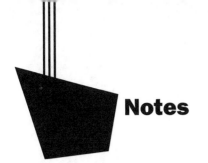

Notes

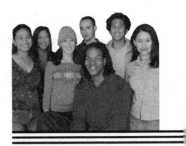

CHAPTER 1

1. E-mail from Joel Newman, United Network for Organ Sharing (UNOS or www.unos.org) June 2004.

2. Ibid.

3. Ibid.

4. www.unos.org (accessed June 2004)

5. www.giftofhope.org/statisticsinformation/qanda.asp (accessed June 2004)

CHAPTER 2

1. www.unos.org (accessed June 2004)

2. www.transweb.org/qu/asktw/answers9702/stomachtransplants.html (accessed June 2004)

3. www.transweb.org/qu/asktw/answers9801/largeintestine.htm (accessed June 2004)

4. www.transplantliving.org/transplant101/gettingOnTheList.asp (accessed June 2003)

5. Newman, June 2004

6. www.unos.org/sitemap.asp (accessed June 2004)

7. www.optn.org/data/ar2002/ar02_table_11010_hr.htm (accessed May 2003)

8. www.unos.org (click on QandA from home page; accessed June 2004)

9. www.unos.org/inTheNews/factsheets.asp (accessed June 2004)

10. www.transplanthealth.com/tt/tt_history02.html (accessed February 2003)

CHAPTER 3

1. Toni Rizzo, "Heart Transplantation," in Donna Olendorf, Christine Jeryan, and Karen Boyden, eds., *Gale Encyclopedia of Medicine,* vol. 3 (Detroit, MI: Gale Group, 1999), 1376. Reprinted by permission of The Gale Group.

2. Ibid.

3. www.giftofhope.org/statisticsinformation/qanda.asp (accessed June 2004)

4. Rizzo, p. 1376

5. Ibid.

6. www.transplanthealth.com/tt/tt_history01.html (accessed June 2003)

7. Rizzo, p. 1376

8. Ibid.

9. Ibid.

10. Ibid.

11. Pamphlet: Life Source, March 2002.

CHAPTER 4

1. www.unos.org (accessed June 2004)

2. "News Service Reports," *The Record* (NJ state newspaper, February 27, 2003).

3. www.liverfoundation.org/cgi-bin/dbs/chapter.cgi?db= newsanduid (The Liver Foundation; accessed May 2003)

4. www.suntimes.com/output/news/28transplant.html (accessed July 28, 2003)

5. www.liverfoundation.org (The Liver Foundation; accessed May 2003)

6. www.liverfoundation.org/db/stories/1006 (The Liver Foundation; accessed May 2003)

7. www.transplanthealth.com/tt/tt_history01.html (accessed June 2003)

8. "The Evaluation of Patients with End-Stage Liver Disease as Candidates for Liver Transplantation," Rush-Presbyterian-St. Luke's Medical Center in Chicago, IL: pamphlet (n.d.)

9. Kimberlee Roth, "Living with Hepatitis: We've Known About A and B, but Watch Out for Sinister C," *Chicago Tribune* (June 9, 2002).

10. www.giftofhope.org/statisticsinformation/qanda.asp (Gift of Hope Organ and Tissue Donor Network; accessed June 2004)

11. http://cancer.mednet.ucla.edu (University of Chicago Hospitals and Health System, online Press Release 2002, regarding UCLA's Jonsson Comprehensive Cancer Center)

CHAPTER 5

1. Paula Anne Ford-Martin, "Kidney Transplantation," in Donna Olendorf, Christine Jeryan, and Karen Boyden, eds., *Gale Encyclopedia of Medicine*, vol. 3 (Detroit, MI: Gale Group, 1999), 1700. Reprinted by permission of The Gale Group.

2. Ibid.

3. Tish Davidson, "Pancreas Transplantation," in Donna Olendorf, Christine Jeryan, and Karen Boyden, eds., *Gale Encyclopedia of Medicine,* vol. 4 (Detroit, MI: Gale Group, 1999), 2149. Reprinted by permission of The Gale Group.

4. www.giftofhope.org/statisticsinformation/qanda.asp (Gift of Hope Organ and Tissue Donor Network; accessed June 2004)

5. Ibid.

6. www.niddk.nih.gov/healt/diabetes/summary/pancisl/pancisl .htm (National Institute of Diabetes and Digestive and Kidney Diseases; accessed June 2003)

7. Ibid.

8. Ford-Martin, p. 1700

9. www.giftofhope.org/statisticsinformation/qanda.asp (Gift of Hope Organ and Tissue Donor Network; accessed June 2004)

10. Ibid.

CHAPTER 6

1. Teresa G. Norris, "Lung Transplantation," in Donna Olendorf, Christine Jeryan, and Karen Boyden, eds., *Gale Encyclopedia of Medicine,* vol. 3 (Detroit, MI: Gale Group, 1999), 1820. Reprinted by permission of The Gale Group.

2. Ibid.

3. www.giftofhope.org/statisticsinformation/qanda.asp (Gift of Hope Organ and Tissue Donor Network; accessed June 2004)

4. Norris, p. 1820

5. www.giftofhope.org/statisticsinformation/qanda.asp (Gift of Hope Organ and Tissue Donor Network; accessed June 2004)

6. Norris, p. 1820

7. Melanie Apel, *Cystic Fibrosis: The Ultimate Teen Guide* (Lanham, MD: Scarecrow Press, Inc., forthcoming).

8. Dinitia Smith, "Battling Failing Health, in Her Own Words" *New York Times,* The Arts, YNE, B1, August 5, 2002.

9. "Alpha-1 Association: Alpha-1 Antitrypsin Deficiency," Minneapolis, MN, 2001; pamphlet; also visit the website at www.alphaone.org (Alpha-1 Association)

CHAPTER 7

1. www.giftofhope.org/statisticsinformation/qanda.asp (Gift of Hope Organ and Tissue Donor Network; accessed June 2004)

2. www.kidney.org/recips/livingdonors/infoQA.cfm (National Kidney Foundation; accessed June 2004)

3. www.giftofhope.org/statisticsinformation/qanda.asp (Gift of Hope Organ and Tissue Donor Network; accessed June 2004)

CHAPTER 8

1. www.trioweb.org/resources/scholarships_c.html (Transplant Recipients International Organization, Inc.; accessed June 2003)

2. http://my.webmd.com/content/pages/7/1809_50990.htm? (accessed February 2004)

3. www.transweb.org/webcast/winter2001/medial.html (accessed June 2003)

4. www.kidney.org/recips/athletics/04games/ (National Kidney Foundation; accessed June 2003)

5. www.unos.org/news/newsDetail.asp?id=243 (United Network for Organ Sharing; accessed June 2003)

CHAPTER 9

1. www.mottep.org/stats.shtml (National Minority Organ Tissue Transplant Education Program; accessed June 2003)

2. www.mottep.org (National Minority Organ Tissue Transplant Education Program; accessed June 2003)

3. www.nationalmottep.org/about.shtml (National Minority Organ Tissue Transplant Education Program; accessed June 2003)

4. Kathy Roth, "Living With Hepatitis; We've Know About A and B, but Watch Out for Sinister C." *Chicago Tribune*, June 9, 2002.

5. www.mottep.org/stats.shtml (National Minority Organ Tissue Transplant Education Program; accessed June 2003)

6. Paul H. Johnson, "Heroes Wanted: Black Doctors Cite a Critical Shortage of Black Organ Donors," *The Record* (NJ state paper, March 16, 2004).

7. www.mottep.org/stats.shtml (National Minority Organ Tissue Transplant Education Program; accessed June 2003)

8. Ibid. [Diabetes Source: American Diabetes Association]

9. Ibid. [Health, US, 2000: American Heart Association; National Vital Statistics Reports, Vol. 48 No. 11]

10. www.mottep.org/stats.shtml (National Minority Tissue Transplant Education Program; accessed June 2003)

11. Ibid. [compliments of UNOS/OPTN Data as of April 4, 2004]

12. E-mail from Abby Hines, American Lung Association, June 2004. (www.lungusa.org)

13. Peter A. Brown, "Troubling Aftermath of a Tragedy," *The Record* (NJ state paper, August 5, 2002).

CHAPTER 10

1. www.sos.state.il.us/biography/biography.html (Illinois Secretary of State; June 2003)

2. www.cyberdriveillinois.com/press/release/030407d1.html (Illinois Secretary of State; June 2003)

3. www.giftofhope.org/dfr/deardonor.asp (Gift of Hope Organ and Tissue Donor Network; June 2003)

4. www.unos.org/Newsroom/archive_newsrelease_20020628_incentives.htm (United Network for Organ Sharing; June 2002)

5. www.donorfoundation.org (June 2004, under construction)

6. www.unos.org (Organ Procurement and Transplantation Network: part of United Network for Organ Sharing, accessed June 2003)

7. www.giftofhope.org/kids/donorman.asp (Gift of Hope Organ and Tissue Donor Network; June 2003)

8. www.mandypatinkin.net/ARTICLES/cornea01.shtml (June 2004)

9. www.pathology.med.miami.edu/btb/mission.html (June 2003)

10. Ibid.

11. E-mail from Reg Green, The Nicholas Green Foundation (www.nicholasgreen.org), June 2004.

12. www.NicholasGreen.org (The Nicholas Green Foundation; June 2003)

13. Green, June 2004.

14. www.giftofhope.org (Gift of Hope Organ and Tissue Donor Network; June 2003)

CHAPTER 11

1. www.unos.org/newsroom/myth_main.htm (United Network for Organ Sharing; accessed June 2002)

2. Galina Espinoza, Karen Brailsford, and Frances Kinkelspiel, "Circle of Life," *People Magazine* (January 14, 2002), 46–51.

3. Cheryl Wittenauer, AP, "Woman Gives Sister Ovary," *The Press Journal* (NJ Paper, April 23, 2004), p. A17

4. www.moviewavs.subportal.com/health/Health_Biz/Therapy_Procedures/organ_transplants (accessed July 2003)

5. www.azcentral.com/offbeat/articles/0701WombTransplants 01-ON.html (accessed July 2003)

6. www.cbsnews.com/stories/2002/12/02/60II/main531402. shtml (accessed June 2002)

7. Catherine Saint Louis, "Family Scars, Three People in Desperate Need of Kidneys, and the Siblings Who Provided Them." *New York Times Magazine* (May 5, 2002), pp. 52–55.

8. www.liverfoundation.org (accessed July 2004).

9. Barbara Powell, AP, "Dr. James Hardy; Performed First Animal-Human Transplant, '64 Surgery Used Chimpanzee Heart" *The Record* (NJ state paper, February 21, 2003), p. L-12, Obituaries.

10. www.msnbc.com/news/878794.asp (accessed March 2003)

11. www.abcnews.go.com/sections/scitech/DailyNews/ clonedpigsstudy020103.html (accessed July 2003)

12. www.msnbc.com/news/878794.asp (accessed March 2003)

13. www.cbsnews.com/stories/2003/02/18/health/main540907 .shtml (accessed April 2003)

14. www.kidney.org/recips/athletics/02games/index.cfm (accessed July 2002)

15. Ibid.

16. http://atheism.about.com/library/weekly/aa052302a.htm (accessed June 2003)

17. www.princeton.edu/pr/pwb/02/1209/1c.shtml (accessed March 2003)

18. E-mail from Joel Newman, United Network for Organ Sharing (UNOS or www.unos.org) June 2004

CHAPTER 12

1. GK, "Hand Transplant Recipient Throws in the Towel," *The Hastings Center Report,* January 2001, vol. 31, il p. 6.
2. Denise Grady, "Kimberly Miles, 33, Recipient in a Rare Lung Transplant," *The Record* (NJ state paper, May 16, 2002).
3. www.alphaone.org (Alpha-1 Foundation; accessed June 2003)
4. Ibid.
5. Ibid.
6. Mary Amoroso, "Son's Story Lovingly Preserved." *The Record* (NJ state paper, May 19, 2002)
7. Janelle London, "People Profiles, Transplantation Changing Lives," www.patients.unos.org/people_1999_05.htm (accessed June 2002)
8. James M. DuBois, "Transplant Error Can Be Prevented," *The Record* (NJ state paper, February 21, 2003).

CHAPTER 13

1. Chuck Nowlen and Tom Alesia, "Doctor Wears a Crown," *Wisconsin State Journal*, June 23, 2003 (www.madison.com/captimes/news/stories/547.php_accessed June 2003)
2. www.kidneyfla.org/p_publiced.html (accessed March 2003)
3. www.mottep.org/n_nmdad.shtml (accessed July 2004)
4. www.trioweb.org/resources/united_c.html (accessed June 2003)
5. www.giftofhope.org/kids/funquiz.asp (accessed June 2003)

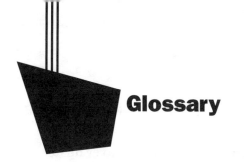

Glossary

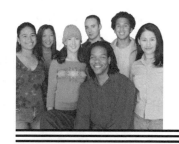

ABO typing The process of classifying human blood into four groups: A, B, AB, and O.

Accelerated rejection The rejection of an organ by the recipient, which occurs 3 to 4 days after surgery. (Accelerated rejection is usually seen in recipients who have had a pervious transplant.)

Acute rejection The rejection of a transplanted organ between 5–90 days after surgery.

Adverse reaction A side effect or reaction from a drug.

Allocation A system designed to ensure that organs are given to recipients in a fair manner.

Antibody A protein made by the body's immune system to fight foreign matter like a virus, bacteria, or even a new organ.

Antigens A protein marker on the surface of cells that tells the body "self or nonself" for each organ (like skin or kidney). It is like a red flag to show something as a "nonself" so that the body will produce antibodies to try and destroy the foreign matter.

Antirejection drugs Medicines that help slow down the body's immune system so it doesn't attack the new "foreign" organ in the body. These drugs are also called "immunosuppressants."

BMX Bicycle motocross is an extreme sport (that takes place all year 'round with outdoor *and* indoor tracks), where riders race around a dirt track made up of huge hills, jumps, and berms. Riders range from 3 years old through

50- or 60-year-olds, whoever can ride a two-wheeler and
wants to race.

BUN (blood-urea-nitrogen) A blood test used to evaluate
renal (which refers to the kidneys) function.

Cardiopulmonary bypass A heart/lung machine that is used
to keep the blood circulating throughout the body while
bypassing, or not using, the actual heart and lungs. The
machine, which keeps the person alive during the
transition, is used while exchanging the diseased organs
for new, healthy ones.

Chronic A disease that develops slowly and lasts for a lengthy
period of time.

Chronic rejection The process in which the body rejects a
transplanted organ 3 months or later posttransplantation.
All transplant recipients worry about chronic rejection.

Cor pulmonale Right heart failure, also called *right ventricular
hypertrophy*, where the right ventricle is damaged and the
blood flow is interrupted. The right ventricle is responsible
for sending oxygen-poor blood to the lungs for oxygen
renewal. Cor pulmonale could be a result of pulmonary
hypertension

Creatinine A substance found in the blood that is used as a
measure to determine how the kidneys are working.

Crossmatch A blood test to see if a donor's organ is a good
match for a body. A negative crossmatch means that there
is no reaction between the patient and the donor, so the
transplant can be performed. A positive crossmatch shows
that the donor and patient are incompatible, so a
transplant should not be performed.

Delayed graft function This occurs when the new organ
doesn't start working immediately after the surgery. Many
kidneys do not function right away after a transplant. The
patient might require dialysis until the kidney starts to make
urine on its own and also sees a decrease in the serum
creatinine.

Diabetes A disease in which patients have high levels of sugar
in their blood that can lead to kidney failure.

Dialysis A therapy that replaces the function of the kidneys by
filtering fluids and waste products out of the bloodstream.

Donor A person who gives an organ to be transplanted into someone else, who is usually referred to as the recipient.

Duodenum The section of the small intestine located immediately after the stomach.

Echocardiogram A medical test that takes ultrasound waves, similar to those used to see a baby in a woman's uterus, to record and show the position and motion of the walls of the heart.

Edema A description for the medical condition in which a body retains excess fluids. Swollen ankles are common signs of edema.

Electrocardiogram A test used to check function of the ventricles in the heart.

Endomyocardial biopsy A medical test in which doctors take a small sample of heart tissue to look for signs of damage caused by organ rejection.

End-stage heart failure A condition in which heart disease has become so severe that no medical or surgical treatments will keep a patient alive.

End-stage organ disease A disease affecting an organ that eventually leads to failure of that organ.

End-stage renal disease (ESRD) A disease or disorder that damages the kidneys so they cannot adequately remove fluids and wastes from the body. The kidneys cannot maintain the proper level of certain chemicals in the bloodstream. Without long-term dialysis or a kidney transplant, ESRD becomes deadly.

Experimental treatment Any new medications, procedures, or treatments that are not yet covered by insurance companies or are not yet approved by the Food and Drug Administration (FDA).

Foreign body Any organ or tissue that is not from the person's body originally. The body will always try to attack such material.

Glomerular filtration rate A measurement of how the kidneys are working that is used to determine the severity of kidney disease.

Glucagon A hormone produced by the pancreas that causes the liver to release its stored sugar into the bloodstream.

Graft pancreatitis Inflammation of the transplanted pancreas.

Graft survival A term known as the percentage of patients who have functioning, transplanted organs. It is usually given as a percentage in 1-, 3-, and 5-year intervals.

Harvest A technical term for removing an organ or tissue by a surgical procedure, to transplant into a sick patient waiting for a healthy organ. This term has been replaced and is more commonly called "recovery" now.

Hemorrhage The loss of large amounts of blood.

HLA system Human leukocyte antigen system. It is a guide that doctors use to determine if another person's genetic makeup will accept an organ from a certain person/possible donor.

Hyperacute rejection The rejection of a transplanted organ within minutes or hours after the transplantation to the recipient. This is the fastest form of rejection.

Immunity The body's ability to resist a particular infectious disease.

Immunosuppressive drug Medication(s) used to lower a patient's immune system (which is like an alarm that triggers the body to fight off infection or foreign cells, like an organ from another body) to lower the risk of rejection.

Incision A cut made to open the skin and abdomen to remove the sick organs and replace them with healthy ones.

Kidneys Two organs responsible for processing water into the body, cleaning the blood, and making urine. A kidney may be donated from a living donor.

Nephrectomy The surgical procedure to remove a kidney from a living donor.

Nonfunction A condition in which the transplanted organ does not function in the body.

Organ A part of the body made of specific and distinctive cells and tissues that perform a particular function (i.e., cardiac cells make up the heart).

Pancreas An organ that produces chemicals that aid in digestion.

Panel reactive antibody (PRA) A medical procedure in which cells taken from potential donors are tested with the recipient's cells to determine the reaction. The more antibodies in a recipient's blood, the more likely the recipient will react against the potential donor. The higher the PRA percentage value, the greater the chance an organ will be rejected.

Pulmonary A term that refers to the breathing function and system (also called the *respiratory system*).

Pulmonary hypertension A rare disease with less than 100,000 patients in the United States. (The number of patients is increasing steadily and if this disease goes untreated, in can become quickly fatal.) [Source: www.pulmonary-hypertension-treatments.com]

Recipient A person who receives a tissue or organ from a donor.

Reflux nephropathy Damage caused to internal structures of the kidney, caused by the backup of urine into the kidney.

Reflux pancreatitis A back flow of urine into the pancreas, causing an inflammation of the pancreas.

Rejection The body's process of attacking and trying to destroy a foreign object, such as germs or a transplanted organ.

Retransplant Transplantation of a second organ after the first organ fails or is rejected.

Sarcoidosis A chronic disease with unknown cause that involves formation of nodules in bones, skin, lymph nodes, and lungs.

Silicosis A progressive disease that results in impairment of lung function and is caused by inhaling dust that contains silica.

Status A code, or level, that is assigned to a patient awaiting a transplant.

Survival rates Rates that indicate the percentage of patients who are alive or grafts that are functioning after a period of time.

Transplant center A medical center that performs organ and/or tissue transplants.

United Network for Organ Sharing (UNOS) An organization that sets policy for transplantation and is involved with assisting centers with matching, transplantation, and sharing of organs.

Ureter A vessel that transports urine to the bladder from the kidneys.

Waiting list After being medically and psychologically evaluated as an accepted candidate for organ transplant, the patient is placed on a national waiting list for organs. When an organ becomes available, the UNOS computer generates a list of potential recipients based on genetic similarities, blood type, organ size, medical urgency, and time that the recipient has been on the list.

Xenotransplant A transplant of animal tissues into humans.

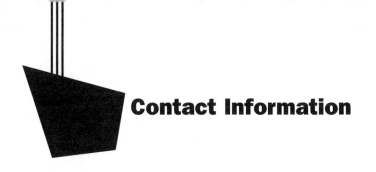

Contact Information

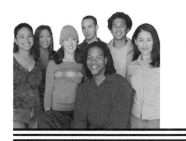

WEBSITES

BMX Racing

www.ababmx.com (American Bicycle League)
www.nbl.org (National Bicycle League)

Donation

www.redcross.org/donate/tissue (American Red Cross Tissue
    Donation)
www.anatomicgift.com/banks.cfm (Anatomic Gift Foundation)
http://medschool.umaryland.edu/programs/BTBank/ (Brain and
    Tissue Bank for Developmental Disorders—University of
    Maryland)
www.core.org (Center for Organ Recovery and Education—
    CORE)
www.organdonor.gov (U.S. Department of Health and Human
    Services)
www.whareyourlife.org (Coalition on Donation)
www.donors1.org (Gift of Life Donor Program, re: tissues)
www.marrow.com (National Marrow Donor Program)

Donor Families

www.aarp.org/griefandloss (AARP: Coping with grief and loss)
www.angelfire.com/ms/DonorMoms (Anglefire: A Place for
    Donor Moms, FYI: web address is case sensitive)

www.compassionatefriends.org (Compassionate Friends: Grief Support After the Death of a Child)

www.griefworks.com (Griefworks)

www.journeyofhearts.org (Journey of Hearts)

www.kidsplace.org/index.html (The Kids' Place, children and grief)

Financial Aid and Fundraising Sites

www.cota.org (Children's Organ Transplant Association—Provides fundraising assistance for children needing life-saving transplants and promotes organ, marrow, and tissue donation)

www.hcfa.gov (Health Care Financing Administration)

www.Transplantfund.org (National Transplant Assistance Fund)

General Transplant Websites (to answer all questions)

www.redcross.org/tissue (American Red-Cross Tissue Services)

www.a-s-t.org (American Society of Transplantation)

www.americantransplant.org (American Transplant Association)

www.americantransplant.org/transplant_glossary.htm (American Transplant Organization)

www.geocities.com/otsfriends (Organ Transplant Support, Inc.)

www.hhs.gov (U.S. Dept. of Health and Human Services)

www.mayo.edu (Mayo Clinic in Minneapolis, MN)

www.nationalmottep.org (National Minority Organ and Tissue Transplantation Education Program)

www.nicholasgreen.com

www.transplant-speakers.org (Transplant Speakers International)

www.transplanthealth.com (Transplant Health)

www.transplantation-soc.org (Transplantation Society)

www.transweb.org/reference_sites/centers.htm (Transplant Web Organization) www.trioweb.org (Transplant Recipient International Organization)

www.unos.org (United Network for Organ Sharing)

www.webmd.org (World Wide Web Medical Doctor Organization)

Heart Information

www.americanheart.org (American Heart Association)

www.heartinfo.org (Heart Info.Org)

www.health-heart.org (Health-Heart.org—Tips on How to Have a Healthy Heart)

www.nhlbi.nih.gov/chd/ (National Heart, Lung and Blood Institute; National Institute of Health)

Illinois Organizations (You can check your own state for various sites like these)

www.cyberdriveillinois.com (Illinois' Secretary of State Website; leading state for Organ donation)

www.giftofhope.org (Gift of Hope Organ and Tissue Donor Network)

www.illinoiseyebank.org (Illinois Eye-Bank)

www.illinois-liver.org (IL Chapter of American Liver Foundation)

www.sos.state.il.us/grograms/programs_organ.htm (IL Secretary of State)

Kidney, Pancreas, and Islet Information

www.childrenwithdiabetes.org (Children with Diabetes)

www.diabetes.org (American Diabetes Foundation)

www.diabetesliving.org (part of www.DiabetesPortal.com which links to 14 websites, used in 35+ countries around the world!)

www.insulinfree.org (Insulin-Free World Foundation)

www.islet.org (The Islet Foundation)

www.jdrf.org (Juvenile Diabetes Research Foundation International—JDFI) www.niddk.nih.gov (National Institute of Diabetes, Digestive and Kidney Diseases—NIDDK)

www.kidney.org (National Kidney Foundation)

www.insulinfreetimes.org (National Pancreas and Islet Transplant Association)

www.worldkidneyfund.org (World Kidney Fund)

Kids' Sites

www.KidsKare.org (Kids Kare)

www.donors1.org/kids/donorsaurs2.html (Gift of Life Program)

Liver Information

www.liverfoundation.org (American Liver Foundation)

www.cdc.gov/ncidod/diseases/hepatitis/index.htm (Centers for Disease Control and Prevention)

www.my.webmd.com/condition_center_hub/hep (WebMD Hepatitis Center)

www.HepatitisMag.com (Hepatitis Magazine)

Lung Information

www.alpha1.org (Alpha1 Association)

www.cff.org (Cystic Fibrosis Foundation)

www.lungUSA.org (American Lung Association)

www.lunglifecenter.com (Lung Life Center)

www.2ndwind.org (Second Wind)

www.ishlt.org (ISHLT: The International Society for Heart and Lung Transplantation)

Pharmacies/Directories

www.transplantrx.com (The Transplant Pharmacy)

www.goodliferesources.com (Goodlife Resources)

www.lifelinkfound.org/pharmacy.html (LifeLink Transplant Institute)

Television Websites to Search for Latest Media Stories (Re: Transplantation/Organ Donation)

www.abcnews.go.com
www.cbsnews.com/stories/2002/12/02/60II/main531402
   .shtml
www.cnn.com/health
www.msnbc.com/news
www.fox.com

ORGANIZATIONS

AirLifeLine
AirLifeLine National Office
50 Fullerton Court, Suite 200
Sacramento, CA 95825
Toll Free: 877-AIR-LIFE
(916) 641-7800
www.airlifeline.org
This is a national nonprofit organization of over 1,500 private pilots who fly ambulatory patients who cannot afford the cost of travel to medical facilities for diagnosis and treatment. Our pilots donate their time, aircraft, and fuel to make this air transportation service totally free of charge for patients who qualify.

American Association of Kidney Patients (AAKP)
3505 E. Frontage Road, Suite 315
Tampa, FL 33607
1-800-749-2257
www.aakp.org

American Diabetes Foundation
National Center
1701 N. Beauregard Street
Alexandria, VA 22311
1-800-DIABETES (1-800-342-2383)
www.diabetes.org

American Heart Association
National Center
7272 Greenville Avenue
Dallas, TX 75231
1-800-242-8721
www.americanheart.org

American Kidney Fund (AKF)
6110 Executive Blvd., Suite 1010
Rockville, MD 20852
800-638-8299
www.akfinc.org
This organization provides limited grants to needy dialysis and kidney transplant patients and living kidney donors to help with costs of transplantation, medicine, and other treatment needs.

American Liver Foundation (ALF)
75 Maiden Lane, Suite 603
New York, NY 10038
1-800-Go-Liver (1-800-465-4837) or 1-888-4HEP-USA (1-888-443-7872)
www.liverfoundation.org

American Lung Association
61 Broadway, 6th Floor
New York, NY 10006
(212) 315-8700
www.lungUSA.org

American Organ Transplant Association
3335 Cartwright Road
Missouri City, TX 77459
(281) 261-2682
This is an organization that assists organ transplant recipients defray out-of-pocket expenses. Provides fundraising assistance and reduced-cost or free transportation to transplant patients and their families.

American Transplant Association (Patient-Oriented Education,
Services and Support)
980 N. Michigan Avenue, Suite 1400
Chicago, IL 60611
1-800-494-4527
E-mail: ata@americantransplant.org

Association of Organ Procurement Organizations
1364 Beverly Road, Suite 100
McLean, VA 22101
www.aopo.org

Brain and Tissue Bank for Developmental Disorders
University of Maryland, Baltimore
Department of Pediatrics
Room 10-035 BRB
655 W. Baltimore Street
Baltimore, MD 21201-1559
1-800-847-1539
E-mail: btbumab@umaryland.edu
http://medschool.umaryland.edu/programs/BTBank/

Cystic Fibrosis Foundation
6931 Arlington Road
Bethesda, MD 20814
800-FIGHT CF (344-4823)
E-mail: info@cff.org
http://www.cff.org

Fujisawa Patient Assistance Program
800-477-6472
This program helps patients with the costs of
immunosuppressant drugs.

HRSA Division of Transplantation
Health Resources and Service Administration
U.S. Department of Health and Human Services
Parklawn Building

5600 Fishers Lane
Rockville, MD 20857
www.hrsa.gov/osp/dot

LifePage
Customer Care:
1-877-265-UCOM (8266)
E-mail: customercare@UCOM.com
www.nepaging.com/lifepage.htm

Musculosketal Transplant Foundation (MTF-Changing Lives
Through Tissue Donation)
125 May Street
Edison, NJ 08837
E-mail: Information@mtf.org
www.MTF.org

National Donor Family Council (part of www.kidney.org/
recips/donor/)
800-622-9010

National Kidney Foundation (NKF)
30 East 33rd Street, Suite 1100
New York, NY 10016
1-800-622-9010

National Transplant Assistance Fund (NTAF)
3475 W. Chester Pike, Suite 230
Newtown Square, PA 19073
1-800-642-8399
E-mail: NTAF@transplantfund.org

The Nicholas Green Foundation
P.O. Box 937
Bodega Bay, CA 94923
E-mail: green@sonic.net
www.nicholasgreen.org

Transplant Speakers International, Inc.
P.O. Box 6395
Freehold, NJ 07728
Toll free (877) 609-4615
Fax 732 577 1003

TRIO (Transplant Recipient International Organization, Inc.)
2117 L Street, NW, #353
Washington, DC 20037
1-800-TRIO-386
E-mail: triointl@aol.com

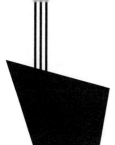

Suggested Reading

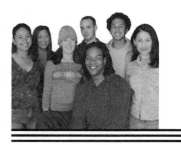

Finn, Robert. *Organ Transplants: Making the Most of Your Gift of Life*. Beijing; Sebastopol, CA: O'Reilly and Associates, Inc., 2000.

Fringuello, Judy. *Tim's Place*. Emerson, NJ: Nu Leaf Publishing, 2002.

Fullick, Ann. *Rebuilding the Body: Organ Transplantation*. Chicago, IL: Heinemann Library, 2002.

Green, Reg. *The Nicholas Effect: A Boy's Gift to the World*. Sebastopol, CA: O'Reilly and Associates, 1999. (www.nicholasgreen.org)

Gutkind, Lee. *Many Sleepless Nights: The World of Organ Transplantation*. New York, NY: W.W. Norton, 1988.

Murphy, Wendy B. *Spare Parts: From Peg Legs to Gene Splices*. Brookfield, CT: Twenty-First Century Books/The Millbrook Press, 2001.

Myers, Edward. *When Will I Stop Hurting? Teens, Loss, and Grief: The Ultimate Teen Guide*. (It Happened to Me, No. 8). Lanham, MD: Scarecrow Press, 2004.

———. *Coping Effectively: A Guide for Patients and Their Families*. National Kidney Foundation. (n.d.). (To order, call toll free 1-800-622-9010).

Parr, Elizabeth. *I'm Glad You're Not Dead: A Liver Transplant Story* (2nd ed.). N.p.: Journey Publishing, 2000.

Parr, Elizabeth, and Janet Mize. *Coping With an Organ Transplant, Sound Information and Meaningful Advice from an Organ Transplant Recipient and a Transplant Nurse*. New York: Avery/Penguin Putnam, 2001.

———. *What Every Patient Needs to Know*. Richmond, VA: United Network for Organ Sharing, 2004. (To order, call toll free 1-888-TXINFO-1)

Picoult, Jodi. *My Sister's Keeper*. New York: Atria Books, April 2004.

Rothenberg, Laura. *Breathing for a Living*. New York: Hyperion Press, July 2003.

Tilney, Nicholas L. *Transplant: From Myth to Reality*. New Haven, CT: Yale University Press, 2003.

Walton, Karen A., and with Allison Patrice Peterson, Illustrator. *How Will They Get that That Heart Down Your Throat? A Child's View of Transplants*. N.p.: E.M. Press, 1999.

Winters, Adam. *Organ Transplants: The Debate Over Who, How, and Why*. New York: The Rosen Publishing Group, 2000.

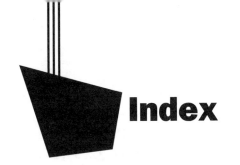

Index

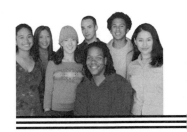

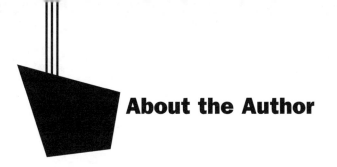

About the Author

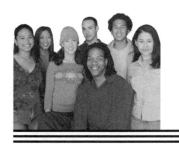

Tina P. Schwartz lives in Grayslake, Illinois, with her husband Marc and their three children. She writes books for children and young adults. Her father, Jim, had a liver transplant in 1995 that saved his life and allowed him to live to see her children be born and watch them grow. Mrs. Schwartz does author visits and gives writing seminars at schools and libraries all over the country. She is a self-proclaimed tomboy who enjoys playing sports and going to the movies, and she especially likes children and dogs.